Best [illegible]

Jennifer + Dan

[illegible signature]

Despite MS, to Spite MS

Despite MS, to Spite MS

One couple facing the challenges
of life and Multiple Sclerosis

DAN AND JENNIFER DIGMANN

Magee Press | Mount Pleasant, Mich., 2011

Printed in the United States of America

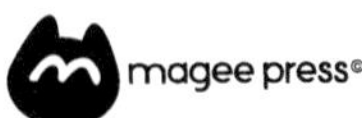

This book is a publication of Magee Press, Mount Pleasant, Mich.

www.danandjenniferdigmann.com
Telephone orders 1-989-775-8475
Online orders @ www.despitemstospitems.com

Cover design by Stacy Simmer. Photo by Ryan Evon.

ISBN 978-0-615-49599-6

Library of Congress Control Number: 2011911874

The paper in this publication meets the minimum requirements of American National Standard for Information Sciences – Permanence of Paper for Printed Library Materials, ANSI Z39. 48–1984

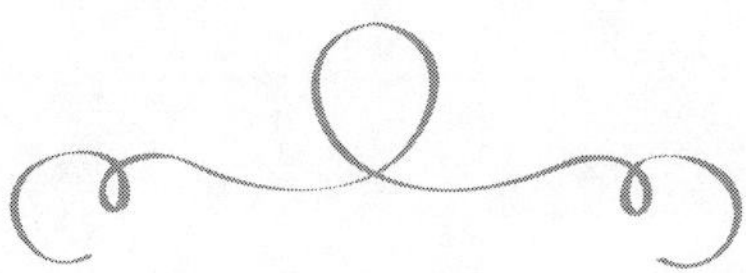

For the more than two million people worldwide
living with Multiple Sclerosis who can relate to our realities,
and for the countless friends and families who help to
strengthen us all in our fight.

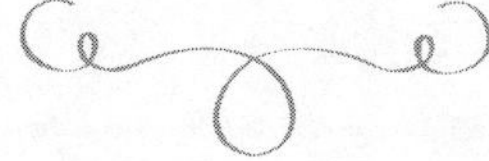

Foreword

As Dan and I began to imagine writing this book, I wondered if there was a real need for it. After all, when you search Amazon.com for books containing the words "Multiple Sclerosis," you'll find more than 2,100 titles. So I wondered if searching "Multiple Sclerosis love stories" or "positive Multiple Sclerosis stories" would generate anywhere near a similar number of titles.

Five.

Yes, five titles came about. And that's after you combine the totals from both searches. So with that bit of unscientific research, I validated what I already knew. Our story needs to be shared. More than that, our daily accounts of life with MS need to be told.

Not only does our story need to be told, but our voices should be heard. Mine being that of a woman living life with MS and a wheelchair, being as hopeful and positive as possible, Despite MS. And, the voice of a man, my husband, who is working, running, and also living a hopeful and positive life, to Spite MS.

While our life isn't easy and we are ALWAYS aware of our Multiple Sclerosis, we hope by sharing our stories we can comfort, educate and inspire you no matter what challenges you are facing.

Jennifer Digmann

Contents

Contents

Acknowledgments

We remember what it was like when we were first diagnosed with Multiple Sclerosis. We were full of questions and fears of how it would affect us. Real, positive stories from the people who had been there, done that and were still moving forward encouraged us to do the same. We pray and hope our stories of living with MS serve as similar voices of reassurance to others.

Our book was developed using various blog-inspired essays we each have written since being diagnosed, and we organized them by specific themes rather than chronological order. And being mindful of the visual difficulties this disease can cause, we chose to publish it in a large-text format.

We are grateful to the countless people who have supported us throughout our lives in dealing with and staying emotionally ahead of MS. We offer heartfelt thanks to our families for their unconditional love, tolerance and patience, and to members of the National MS Society community – especially our groups in Alma, Flint and Mount Pleasant as well as Team MonsterS – for their empowerment and encouragement.

We will forever be indebted to Cynthia Drake and Wesley Leonard for making our nationally recognized blog – danandjenniferdigmann.com – a reality, and thanks to graphic designer Amy Gouin for designing our printed materials and to HealthCentral and to various community agencies and businesses that provided us the opportunities to share our stories and increase MS awareness.

Special thanks to everyone involved in helping to develop this book, including graphic designer (and still our Best Man!) Stacy Simmer; editors Barbara Sutherland Chovanec, Terri Nelson and Mark Lagerwey; instigator Sherene McHenry; publishing advisor Roy Burlington; as well as to photographers Robert Barclay, Brightroom Photography, Peggy Brisbane, Ryan Evon, Ashley Miller and Will Moore for giving us permission to use the photos they've taken of us over the years. And to Judy Williams for allowing us to feature some of the most inspirational haiku-style poems from her blog, *Peace Be With You on the MS Journey*. Peace be with you as well, Judy. Your words move us each day.

Finally to our matchmaker, Karen Bables. Thank you for sparking our first story when you told Dan to sit at Jennifer's table that fateful September day in 2002.

Introduction

I want to tell you about my friends, Dan and Jennifer Digmann.

Dan and Jennifer are a married couple living – thriving, actually – with Multiple Sclerosis, a chronic disease that attacks the central nervous system. It would be easy to look at their lives as a series of struggles, from Dan's numbness and fatigue to Jennifer's inability to walk. But that would be missing the point.

The point is that every day before they have a meal together Dan and Jennifer have a little ritual of clinking forks together and looking into each other's eyes. Or that they complete each other's stories like they're reading from the same script. Or that Jennifer reminds Dan to "pick up your feet" before he goes running every day.

The point is that when Jennifer asked Dan if he ever got tired of helping her use the bathroom, he looked at her, reminded her of the time he drove across the country thinking about how he wanted to marry her more than anything else in the world.

His response to her question? "This is what I prayed for."

I think about that scenario – the idea of feeling such gratitude for the ability to help your spouse with even the most basic everyday needs. It's a position few 20- or 30-somethings would ever imagine themselves in. But it happened to Dan and Jennifer, and their marriage is one of the strongest I've ever known.

Dan and Jennifer have taken their marriage and turned it into what we all wish for our own marriages – a partnership, a presence that makes people want to be better, do better.

Their marriage is an act of activism, a by-any-means-necessary approach to living life with joy and gratitude. They walk, they blog, they raise money, they lobby on the steps of capitol buildings.

And through it all, they embody the spirit of love – that thing I believe we are all destined to be if we shake away the trivialities and talk about what's really important in life. The point is that they make the world a better place, plain and simple. And in doing so they challenge us to reach deep down and do the same thing.

Cynthia J. Drake
January 2011

1

Keeping It Real

I know folks mean well
telling me it is best to
look on the bright side

Sometimes wisdom says,
admit that things are awful.
You got unlucky.

I can be grateful
for gifts this challenge gave me
and still hate MS.

–*JUDY WILLIAMS*

Let me tell you … about my MS wedding

BY DAN

Movie writers would never dream up a fairytale of two people with MS falling in love and living happily ever after.

But Jennifer and I have been living this truest of love stories. We started a new chapter when we were married last year, on September 10, 2005.

MS brought us together

Combined, we've taken on this chronic illness for more than a dozen years. Jennifer was diagnosed eight years ago and claims an unwanted seniority over me by nearly 27 months. She has secondary-progressive MS. Mine is relapsing-remitting.

We met three years ago at a special National MS Society program called "Finding Your Buried Treasure." Jennifer was one of the small group leaders at this daylong program intended to help people with MS rediscover the goals and dreams they'd lost sight of in dealing with the rigors of everyday lives.

How convenient that a National MS Society program manager told me to sit at Jennifer's table. She thought Jennifer and I would have a lot to talk about because we both were younger and were both self-help group leaders.

We wound up talking more about other things: our respective fantasy football teams, how her dog, Buster, had destroyed her Tom Petty hat, and my passion for Bruce Springsteen's music.

I fell in love with Jennifer the day we met. Periodic email messages led to regular telephone calls. But one fateful Thursday night, I received a phone call from her brother, Steve, who told me they had taken Jennifer to the hospital.

Apparently MS felt it wasn't getting enough attention in our relationship.

The next step

That weekend I drove more than 200 miles roundtrip to visit Jennifer in the hospital as she recovered from a severe exacerbation. In the middle of a heart-to-heart conversation about where we thought our relationship was going, she let me know for sure in eight words.

"I think I want you to kiss me," she said as she bit her bottom lip.

Not believing what I had just heard, I sought more direction.

"You mean, like, right now?"

Our relationship took off from there.

Jennifer lived more than 90 minutes away from me, so for nearly three years we spent at least an hour on the phone each weeknight, and I'd make that 200-mile roundtrip to see her each weekend. On October 23, 2004, I asked Jennifer to be my wife.

The main event

Anyone who has ever planned a wedding knows it isn't simple. From caterers and bands to flowers and guest lists, there are so many details. And because most bridal magazines don't specialize in tips for planning accessible weddings, there were a lot of things we had to figure out on our own.

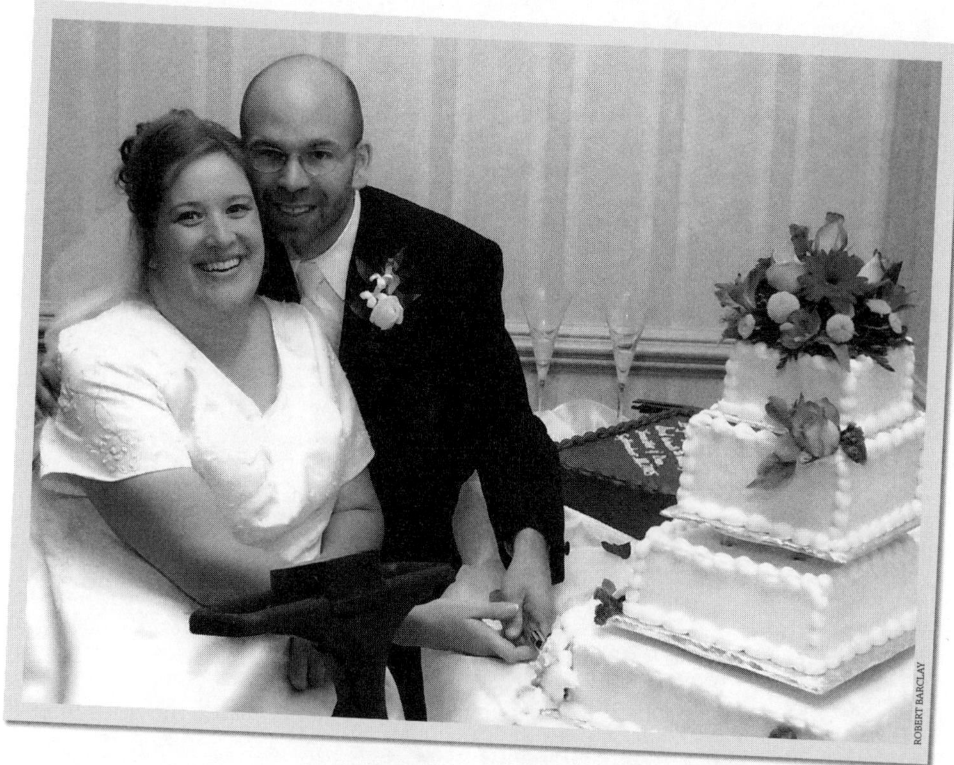
ROBERT BARCLAY

We held our ceremony and reception in the same hotel conference center. This limited scooter-to-van transfers and made things easier for our out-of-town guests and our friends who also have MS.

A late-morning service and early afternoon reception put us all one step ahead of MS-related fatigue, and a jazz quartet playing at the reception added a touch of class. It also thwarted the awkwardness of having to sit out the Hokey Pokey or the Chicken Dance. We avoided a cumbersome buffet line by having a sit-down lunch where wait staff served us all chicken parmesan.

And our honeymoon? We took a weeklong trip to Toronto, where we saw the Blue Jays take on Jennifer's beloved Boston Red Sox.

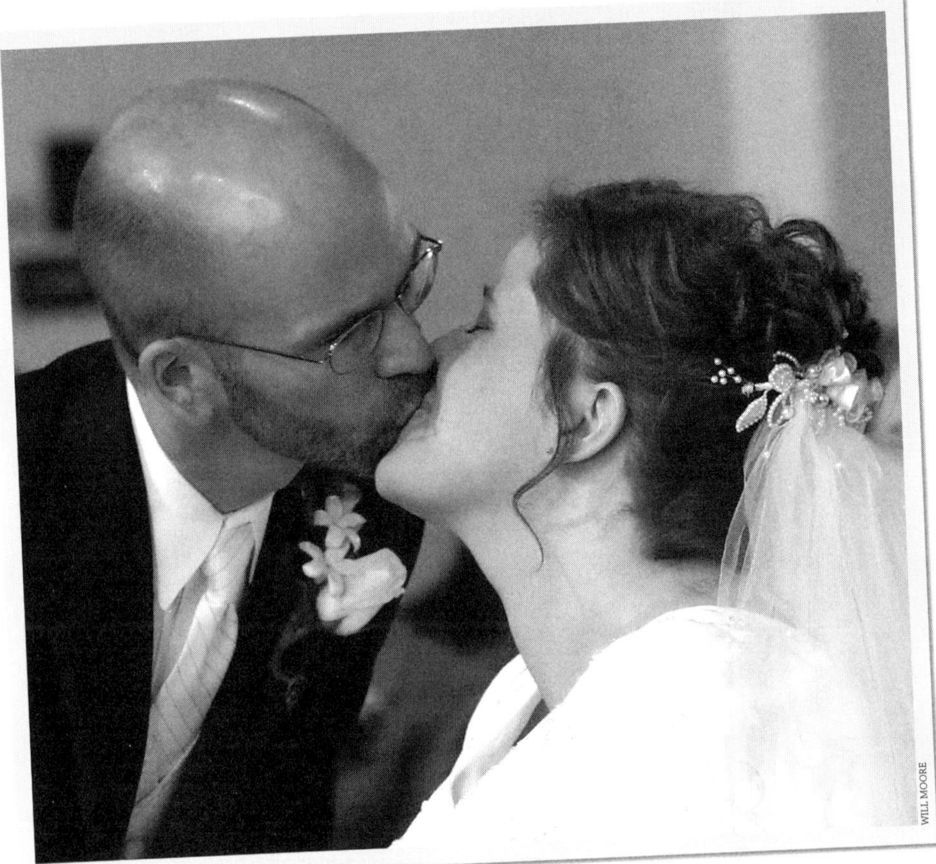
WILL MOORE

From my MS fatigue and constant numbness to Jennifer's spasticity and regular Novantrone treatments, we willingly face every challenge the disease throws at us.

But the MS doesn't define who we are.

And our love story continues ...

This article originally appeared in the membership magazine of the National MS Society (Inside MS).

but i wanted to clean that up!

BY JENNIFER

no, my very first essay will not be about cleaning up our cat, cooper's, pee. it's just that our bundle of joy, as we often call cooper, missing his litter box is one of those little annoyances of life that i miss. believe it or not, i miss being able to clean up cat pee!

i miss it because multiple sclerosis makes it easier for someone else to clean up the mess. after making a genuine offer to help, dan weighed his options: it was either me stooping over the box cursing in frustration or him calmly cleaning up cooper's pee. he chose option 2. and while i don't blame him, i just wish i could have done it. that is what he lives with as my husband as well as my caregiver, damned if you do, damned if you don't.

first off, let me introduce myself, i'm jennifer digmann. i will be occasionally sharing my tales of my daily life with multiple sclerosis. i've been living with ms since 1997. my ms is secondary progressive, and i no longer walk. i use a wheelchair but long for functioning legs each and every day. then again, who among us in a chair doesn't?

my writings – or musings, if you will – will never be capitalized. i'm weak on my left side so i seldom use it and one typically uses his or her left hand to press the shift key to capitalize therefore, i don't. yes, i realize that there are many types of voice-activated typing programs on the market, but i am a soft speaker with a subtle lisp (apparently) who is easily frustrated so i'll stick to my right-hand-index-finger typing method, thank you.

did i mention that i'm stubborn, too? and that i have an amazing husband, dan, who is also dealing with his own case of this miserable disease.

i will try to write honestly. none of us, whether you yourself have ms or you are the caregiver of someone living with this disease, needs a pollyanna version of life with multiple sclerosis. i like to be positive but i am trying to be real. however, i don't want to be a whiner. oy... i just really want to clean up cat pee the way i used to.

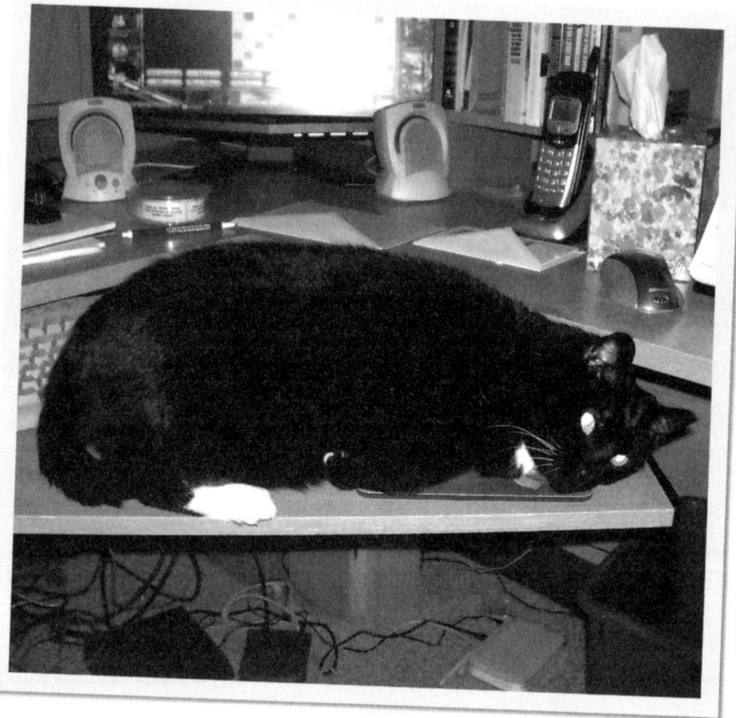

did i do that?

BY JENNIFER

today, i'm feeling quite steve urkel. you know the nerdy, high-waisted jeans and glasses wearing character from the tv show *family matters*. the one with the commonly whined catchphrase, "did i do that?"

i was in my kitchen. i turned to look at something (yeah i can't even remember what, it was that trivial) and then there was a sound – noise more accurately, kind of like nails on chalkboard times 100. this sound was produced by me, naturally. but i have to credit my chair too. it seems that i turned a little too closely next to my refrigerator. my beautiful, surprisingly pristine looking refrigerator.

now, true to form, my refrigerator door is the proud new owner of a decent-sized scratch. and yet again, in my best steve urkel, i am embarrassedly uttering the words, "did i do that?"

this is the risk of living with wheels, or in other words, being in a wheelchair.

as i wrote when describing my bathroom for a correctly capitalized graduate-level english paper earlier this year, "... the absence of crisp, sharp corners on my wooden vanity and towel closet. This demonstrates the fact that I am not a good or careful scooter driver. When one consistently bumps into cabinets or cuts corners a little too closely these are some tell-tale signs."

like the bathroom, my kitchen is a room that has seen its share of damage. damage i thought i would be less likely to create when i started using a power wheelchair, as opposed to the one-woman wrecking machine that was my scooter. but no matter the chair, if i'm driving it, destruction is sure to lie in my path!

well, it looks like i'm going to have to add appliance scratches to my list of tell-tale signs. sorry dan, but all i can do is smile and say, "did i do that?"

Our anniversary ...
me and my mistress in Chicago

BY DAN

As we stroll down Chicago's Christmas-decked Michigan Avenue, you squeeze my hand and remind me that this day is our second anniversary. Not the anniversary that formally solidified our future together, but the anniversary of the day we were introduced.

In these two years you faithfully have been with me every day, and my mind can't stop thinking about you. Thinking about what you do for me each day of my life, and dreaming of what our future holds. Just as parents in some cultures decide on the unions of their children, it was two years ago this day that I first was told that you likely would be with me 'til death do we part.

"The radiologist said the cause of your symptoms most likely is Multiple Sclerosis," my physician told me over the phone at 9:25 a.m. that day, exactly one week from Christmas Eve. Our relationship officially was confirmed by my neurologist on Valentine's Day. What a fitting day to remember the one that will be with you through everything – from here to eternity.

Unconditionally.

But it is our first date that I remember most. How with one telephone call you altered my life. And two years is quite some time for this close a relationship. Granted, we've had our fallouts and spats, but in the end, I'm reminded that you'll never leave me, and I can never leave you. So we deal with it and move on with our life.

While most unions utilize wedding bands to remind the couple of their commitment, you've added a twist to that tradition and have made my hands constantly numb, as though they have fallen asleep. An unwavering reminder that I am yours, you are mine.

We walk amid the noon pedestrian traffic, against the flow. You hamper my strides because you want to go back to our hotel room and spend some time in bed. You think we've done enough for today. You let me go out with some friends for lunch and so far you haven't said too much about me drinking a beer. But I insist on going to the downtown music store in search of rare-to-find Springsteen gems.

We scour the Virgin record store, and much to your delight, we don't find anything worth buying. You hate it when I find good music. It makes you so jealous because if only for a little while, I forget about you and our relationship. I don't know why you worry. I'm not going anywhere.

We meet some friends who are attending the same conference we are. They're walking a little faster than you would like us to, but I remind you that by walking our slower pace, they'll become suspicious of what we have going on together.

I think about how monumental this day is for us and how I want to share the milestone with them, but I know they won't understand. You are like my mistress – I just call you "Ms." And while others know about us, it would make them uncomfortable if I revealed intimate details of our relationship. No one but us can truly appreciate this moment.

One more workshop, and the day's conference activities are over. I convince you that we can go out for a night on the town with my friends. You plead to celebrate the anniversary alone in our room, order some room service, and go to bed early. But I want to go out one last time and make the most of our anniversary.

We go with friends to an Italian restaurant, and I order the Italian sausage dish. And a beer. You didn't do too much to me following my luncheon pilsner, so I anticipate you will lower the boom with excessive fatigue after a Heineken for dinner. But let's be real about this. I am in the mood to order a second beer just to spite you, but it is the price I have to pay the waiter, not you, that keeps me from indulging on our anniversary.

Dinner is over, and we continue visiting with my friends. You're getting anxious to get back to the hotel. All you want to do is get me in bed. But I'm enjoying myself on the town tonight.

I'm so committed to denying you, on the walk back to the hotel, I stand in line for nearly an hour for some cheese-flavored popcorn. Hey, everybody else was waiting in line outside the store, and my friends and I just had to get a taste of this highly sought-after treat. You're like a whiny little kid pulling on my pant leg because you want to go home. You make my feet burn with numbness as I stand in line. "Whatever," I think.

Alas, we make it to the hotel room, and much to your delight, I change into my shorts and T-shirt and pull down the sheets. Finally, you seem content. My hands and feet still are numb because you like to hold a grudge. But you're not making anything else worse.

So we turn off all the lights but one, crawl into bed, and watch Monday Night Football – the Saints against the Rams. You even allow me the energy to stay up for the whole game. That, or my adrenaline has overpowered you because I have two of my fantasy football league players going tonight.

So here's to two years. A constant struggle? No, not constant. But more often than I'd like. I'll admit it: You've made me a better man because you've enabled me to put everything in my life into the proper perspective. And when I can't do that and feel you overtake my will and spirit, I find strength to overpower you through another fantasy in my life: That someday, they'll come and take you away. Let's be honest: I, and nearly half of a million Americans, don't deserve you.

Happy anniversary, Ms.

april 11 … what a glorious day!

BY JENNIFER

did you shower today? kind of personal, yes i know. but did you take a shower today? you probably did. it's kind of like breathing. you just do it and don't really think about it.

that is until you can't do it.

for the first six years that i knew dan, we would make the drive from michigan to monticello, iowa, to celebrate easter with his family. we'd stay three or four days at a hotel conveniently located close to dan's parents house. it was a cute place – clean, a pool, even free pop-tarts at breakfast, and it was pretty accessible.

well, at least for three or four days. but by day five, despite my efforts to wash up in the bathroom sink or go in town to have my hair washed and coiffed, i **needed** to shower.

only problem was that this cute little hotel did not have a roll-in shower, which is a necessity for me because i can no longer stand. so its absence meant that we had to keep our trip short. just a quick visit, and fortunately everyone understood. we were pretty content but our visit always went by way too fast.

however, this year was different. we wanted and needed to stay almost a full week. that meant that we would have to stay at a different hotel. it's not like i could forego a shower for a whole week! we had to find a hotel in a city bigger than monticello. one with a roll-in shower. one twenty-five or thirty minutes from his parents. bye bye pool, pop-tarts and a convenient location.

or so i thought.

but dan had a kind of crazy idea. "see jennifer, there's this camp not very far away from my parents' house. it's a camp that would be accessible. no, really accessible. roll-in shower accessible."

heck, if there was any place in town where i could take a shower, a real shower, i'd be game. to be honest i was a little skeptical, but i was game. so dan made a few phone calls. then we checked out the camp's website and finally, we packed our bags and off to a camp in iowa we went.

camp courageous was no regular camp. it was amazing. beautiful scenery, friendly staff, great rooms and most important, totally equipped with a roll-in shower. in fact, there were six such showers in our cabin. my cup runneth over with cleanliness.

to be exact, april 11 was the day of my first real shower in iowa in over six years. this is why it was such a glorious day!

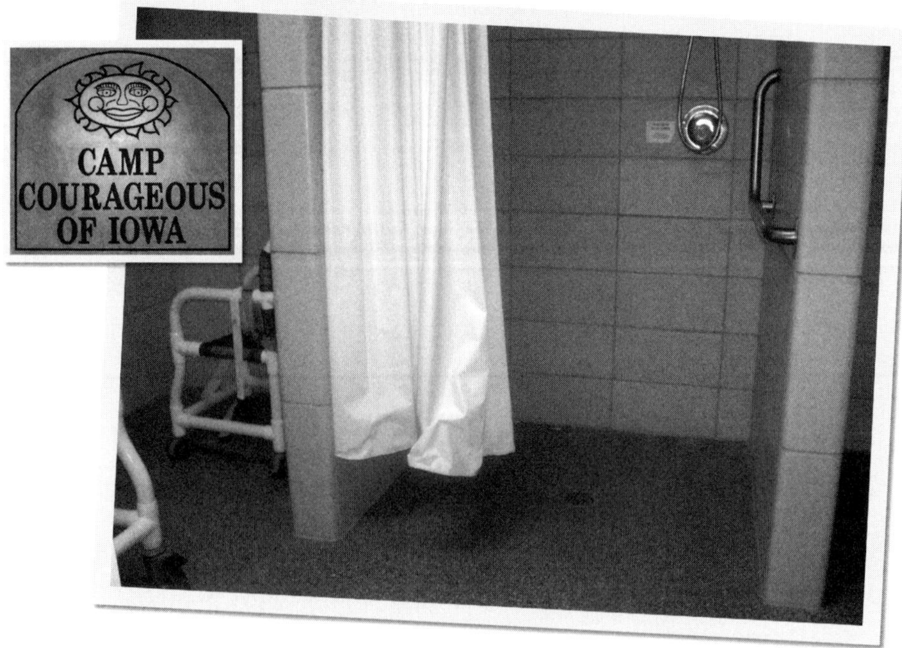

My San Antonio-inspired life

BY DAN

If only I could live every day like I was in San Antonio.

I try, but I sometimes lose sight of the lesson I taught myself in the Lone Star state several years ago.

I was on a three-day business trip, and on the first day there were no conferences or workshops I needed to attend.

So I woke up and, still exhausted from the plane trip, had every intention of spending the entire day in the air-conditioned Red Roof Inn hotel room. I'd eat vending machine food while watching ESPN and take a nap after I had seen the same episode of SportsCenter for the third consecutive time.

After opening my second bag of Doritos to chase the Snickers bar I inhaled for breakfast, the reality of the situation hit me:

Dan, you're in San Antonio. This is your first time here, and you may never make it back again. Go out. Experience it. Live it.

And so I did. Braving the sultry summer San Antonio heat, I went out and took in everything I expected and never expected from this city.

I went to the record store downtown and found four vintage Bruce Springsteen 45 records (and a poster that still hangs in our "Springsteen Room"), took a boat ride along the San Antonio River Walk and saw the Alamodome where my Iowa Hawkeyes often play in the Alamo Bowl.

And of course I toured the Alamo! But unlike Pee Wee Herman, it didn't shock me that there was no basement in the Alamo. It instead floored me that the mission is right in the downtown surrounded by modern buildings. Guess I always thought it was in the middle of the desert.

That evening, I sat near the pool and drank a beer as I reflected on the unforgettable experiences of the day. Thinking of what inspired me to go out in the first place, I was emotionally smacked with a life-altering epiphany:

Why don't I live every day of my life with the same life-embracing attitude I had in San Antonio? From that day forward, I often invoke this San Antonio-inspired outlook on life.

And who'd have thought that one day would be instrumental in helping me deal and cope with the challenges of MS? For all the times I feel like giving up, ignoring opportunities, making excuses, or throwing in the towel, I remind myself:

Dan, you're alive. This is your only time here, and you can never get it back again. Go out. Experience it. Live it.

May all your stars at night be big and bright ...

jenny the dragon slayer

BY JENNIFER

around may 24 i will begrudgingly celebrate a bitter anniversary of sorts. it will mark seven years since i last walked.

you'd think since it has been such a long time, phrases like "i'm going to run to the store," or "let's go for a walk around the neighborhood," would have slowly worked their way out of my lexicon. but no, i say phrases like these just about every day. that's just me, a little blind to my disability maybe or just not hypersensitive to it. these little untruths are not malicious. they are just, well, part of my charm.

inspired by the t.v. show *buffy the vampire slayer*, on tuesday morning i slayed my first dragon. just as dragons incite fear in some, swimming was my fear. so on tuesday, i stared down that beast and i went swimming.

"swimming?" you ask. well, you betcha!

ok, to me swimming is not the breaststroke or the butterfly. it merely is me standing in the swimming pool. for me right now, swimming has become a humongous process that requires the help of three people. well, four if you count the pool lifeguard (i.e. the lift operator). gone are the days of slipping on my suit and diving right in.

the process starts when i ask my husband, dan, to help me put on my suit. we carefully and momentarily stand to adjust it. then he helps me put on some shoes and a sweatshirt, which serves as a cover-up. then, dan passes me off to my caregivers ellie and jim, who drive me to the very accessible pool facility in central

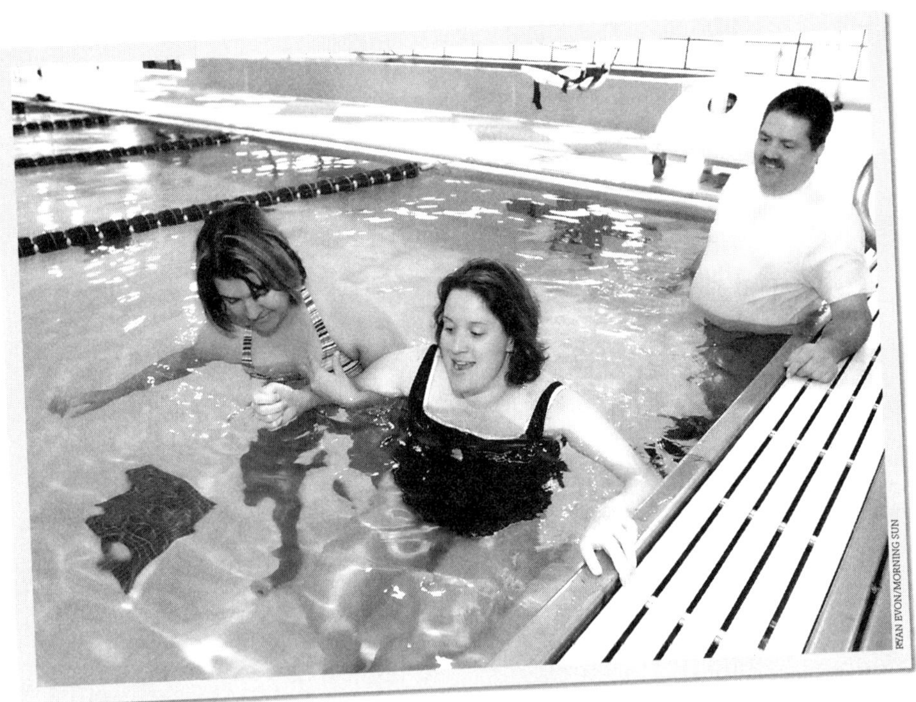
RYAN EVON/MORNING SUN

michigan university's student activity center. ellie escorts me to the locker room where she takes off my cover-up and shoes, hands me my towel and i'm one step closer to taking my swim. oops! see what i mean? i neither step nor swim. again, part of my charm.

once i'm on the pool deck, jim transfers me from my wheelchair to the university's hoyer lift-type thing. and now the lifeguard pushes me, buckled into my seat, close to the water. swimming is so close! i can smell the chlorine and feel the chilly water on my toes. brrr ... finally, i'm submerged up to my chest. time to unbuckle me. oh the water, how refreshing!!

jim floats me over to the stairs, i'll use the handles to position myself. sorry, no miraculous stair climbing in my future. just standing.

ok, wait. **i'm standing!** how amazing is that? because of the water, i'm buoyant and seemingly light as a feather. for me to stand, jim and ellie have to push on my knees to lock them for stability. but once my knees are locked, my caregivers let me go and i'm standing all by myself. for the next 15 minutes, i stand.

as i start to get tired and remember that i don't want to overdo it, i ask jim and ellie to strap me back into the chair, which lifts me up and out of the water. i quietly make a promise to myself that i will swim again this summer. jim transfers me back into my wheelchair, ellie towels me off, and we rush home so i can finally go to the bathroom.

so i went swimming, which is one dragon down. now i have two more i need to overcome. and i'm looking forward to telling you all about them when i finally slay those dragons.

R.I.P. dragons #2 and #3

BY JENNIFER

Taking a graduate class all by myself scared me. There was no Dan to help me or hold my hand. But it actually was an experience that helped me rebuild confidence in my abilities.

Really, it was not that hard. As usual things are much more difficult in my head than they truly turn out to be.

I am sure that I'm not the only person whose confidence has been shaken by this awful disease. My Multiple Sclerosis has tried really hard to take so much away from me and unfortunately, it has won some hard-fought battles. But I've held my ground on this one and didn't let MS win this time.

Since I graduated from college, I have always dreamed of going to graduate school. Marrying Dan, who works for Central Michigan University, made that dream more realistic and possible. I mustered all of my courage and enrolled in a summer session film class. Yes, it lasted only 4 class sessions and was just a 1-credit course, but I signed up and took this class. And not to brag, I didn't just sign up and take it, I ***slayed*** this film class! OK really, I am bragging but for me this is a pretty big accomplishment.

Part of the accomplishment is successfully completing the class and to do this, I had to write papers. Writing class papers was kind of fun and manageable. It was the typing that was difficult. Well it was! With just my right index finger pushing on the keys, it took forever.

But now those days are gone. Well, to be honest and realistic, they are only sort of gone. It's going to take some time and effort to train my new, helpful speak-to-text program, Dragon NaturallySpeaking. I've got plenty of time and a decent amount of patience, and at least it's not my old difficult, almost untrainable program (name rhymes with Mista).

Here's my dragon-slaying record: conquered the pool and, Professor Smith willing, conquered the graduate class. And with a bit of help from a nice dragon, conquered typing. Not just typing, I'm once again typing with capital letters. Did you notice?

That's Jennifer 3, dragons 0. I like that record.

BTW: In case you were wondering, I'm "swimming" tomorrow morning. That'll be the third time since I first told you about slaying my swimming dragon. Oh yeah, and I got an "A" in my graduate film class.

2

Opportunity

The sun rose again.
Gives me opportunity
To define my life.

Do I laugh or cry?
Do I let MS rule me
Or reclaim my life?

I have a choice.
Which life to select for me.
Let me sing and smile.

–*JUDY WILLIAMS*

Kevin Spacey moments

BY JENNIFER

A few years ago I watched a television interview with Kevin Spacey, one of my favorite actors. He has a quiet charm that I find very appealing. Plus, he seems pretty smart, and I think this helps make him a believable actor.

I liked his performance best in the 1999 Oscar-winning film, *American Beauty*. I especially loved it when his character, Lester Burnham, delivered the line, "I'm just an ordinary guy who has nothing left to lose."

Really, haven't we ALL felt like this before? And while I know it's only a line from a character in a movie, I bet Spacey understands this sentiment. But, as usual, I digress. Back to his interview.

In it, Spacey talked about a trip he had taken to Paris or the Great Wall in China, you know, someplace beautiful and historic like that. Anyway, he talks about feeling bad for people who travel to these magnificent sites but are so worried about taking a photo to remember the place or moment that they generally miss experiencing it. He believed that we want so badly to capture these moments in photos that we end up letting them pass us by. His advice was to just put down the camera and live in and enjoy the moments as they happen.

This is great advice I often try to follow. I have repeatedly used my self-coined phrase, "Kevin Spacey moment," to remind me to live in the now. Be there. Enjoy the present. Plus, it makes me feel better when I don't have my camera with me.

Our lunch this past weekend qualified as a "Kevin Spacey moment." Stacy, the best man from Dan's and my wedding, surprised us with a quick visit while he was in town from Indianapolis. The last time we had seen Stacy was when Dan and I went to visit him and his family (and see Dan's favorite, Bruce Springsteen) in March 2008. But this last weekend, not only did we get to see Stacy, we got to see his wife, Heather, and their son, Kieran. I would have loved to have taken a photo to remember their surprise visit, but oops, as usual, no camera.

Instead of pouting because I'd have no photos to remember this visit, I savored our time together talking, laughing and taking plenty of mental pictures. We had a great time, which alas will be remembered as another "Kevin Spacey moment."

So the next time you forget your camera or your batteries aren't charged, remember Kevin Spacey's words to live in and enjoy the moments as they happen. This is great advice to follow even when you have a camera with fully charged batteries.

For You: An open letter to Bruce Springsteen

BY DAN

Dear Bruce Springsteen,

As you scan the sea of signs surrounding the stage that plead for you to play one of your vintage classics at the Palace of Auburn Hills on Nov. 13, my wife, Jennifer, and I won't be there.

Instead, we'll be holding up our "4 U" request all the way across the arena in one of its handicapped-accessible areas. To see us, you gotta look hard.

While we could play the ticket lottery and get our numbers called to stand near the stage the entire concert, our Multiple Sclerosis forces us to stay in our reserved seats.

BRUCE SPRINGSTEEN
4U
NO PARKING
BRUCE SPRINGSTEEN FANS ONLY!
ALL OTHERS WILL BE TOWED

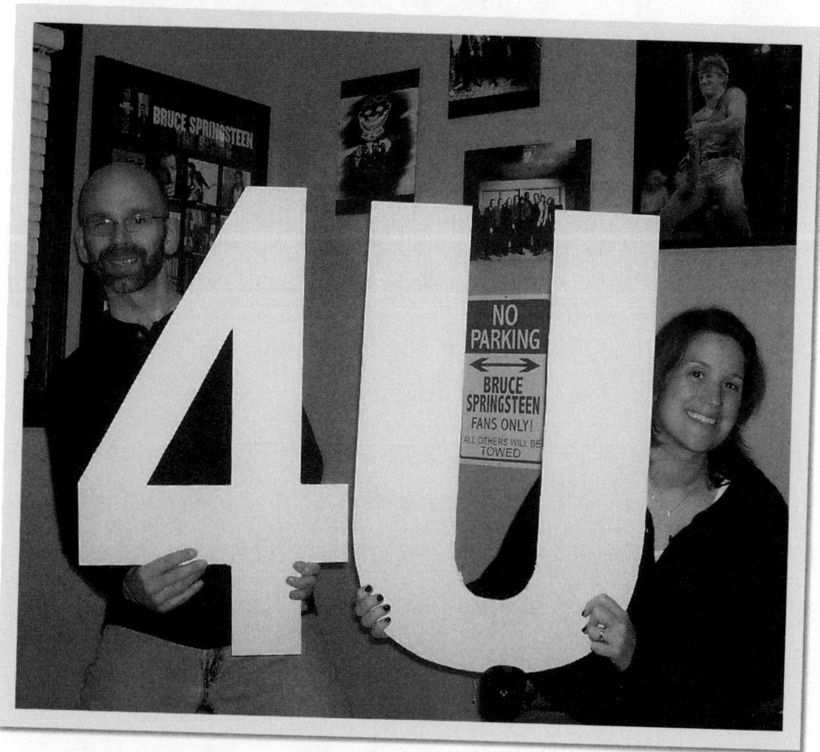

Combined we've had MS for more than 20 years, and we each are living with very different forms of this disease. While I have the relapsing-remitting form and regularly compete in 5K runs, Jennifer has secondary-progressive MS and can no longer walk.

She uses a power wheelchair and this is why we, along with two of our friends coming from Iowa, must stay in the handicapped-accessible area to experience the euphoria that you bring night after night after night after night.

Your music has pulled me through every phase of my life with MS: from fear and self-pity to anger and frustration and finally to acceptance and moving on with the vision of a brighter future. For that, I gratefully thank you.

And if it's not too much to ask you for one favor: When you're searching for requests at the Palace Friday night, please look straight across the arena for my baby and me waving our sign asking you and the E Street Band to play a full-rocking "For You," for us.

All the best,
Dan Digmann
Mount Pleasant, Michigan

BTW: Despite our valiant efforts, Bruce didn't see our sign and play "For You." But no hard feelings. Instead he gave us the entire Born to Run *album. And this marked the last time we'll ever see the E Street Band with saxophonist Clarence Clemons, who passed away June 18, 2011. R.I.P., Big Man. Thanks for sharing your endless gift with us all.*

Goodbye, Jim

BY JENNIFER

Wishing things away is not effective. That's what a fortune cookie once told me. I believe this truism. But knowing this truth didn't stop me from wishing that the news Jim told me a few months ago wasn't true.

Earlier this summer, Jim gently broke it to me that he and his wife were moving to North Carolina. And for as rational as I like to believe myself to be, I started to think that maybe if I wished hard enough he really wouldn't move over 750 miles away.

I am sad because Jim is my main caregiver (next to my husband, Dan, of course). I am eligible for his help because of the MI Choice Medicaid Waiver Program. This program makes it possible for me to continue living with Dan in our own home.

You see, it all started with a simple question from Kathie, the nurse manager in charge of my home care. She and I were at our wits' end after struggling to find a suitable caregiver to help me with my regular activities of daily living. I need help so Dan can continue to work full time, and we'll know I'm getting good care.

Well one day, Kathie asked me if I would be willing to meet her husband to see if he could help me. He wasn't technically "trained" to be a caregiver, but Kathie was hopeful Jim could be the solution for my care, and I was hopeful and really had nothing to lose.

Later that evening, Jim dropped by our house. He met with Dan and me. Almost instantly, we knew this would be a great match. Over the past four years my list of caregivers has included

Diana, Melanie, Leslie, Amy, Libby, Jodi, Kelli, Deb, Ellie and Jen, but my one constant caregiver has been Jim.

He's much more than a caregiver. He's my friend. My fix-it guy. My Detroit Tiger baseball-watching buddy. At times, my savior, and I'm not being dramatic. Sometime I'll tell you the story about getting trapped in our van – a little prison on wheels – from which he rescued me. We cook, our specialty is delicious banana bread. He helps me stretch and motivates me to ride my arm bike – kind of a personal trainer. Also, he's very easy to talk to and share my frustrations with, and he'll give me spiritual insight.

One of the greatest things about him is he's not just help for me. He's made Dan's life easier. He also keeps our cat, Cooper, happy and playful. And he's become a little trivia buddy for my dad.

I'll miss him and all of his help, problem solving and joke telling. But I'm excited to see him move and grab his future. I'm sure he's going to have great success and happiness, but I'm going to miss him. I don't know if I can ever thank him enough. Or if he'll ever know what an impression he has made on me and countless other people in my life.

As Jim was leaving my house his last day as my caregiver, when I started feeling sad about his moving, his parting words to me were, "Remember it's just geography."

That's just like Jim. He's right. While I will no longer see him several days a week, he will only be a phone call away. I am scared that he's leaving, yet I look forward to an exciting future. For him and for me.

Goodbye Jim. God bless you. Good luck in your promising, fantastic future. Thank you from the bottom of my heart.

And we were really dancing

BY DAN

Moving to the music on the dance floor is nothing new for Jennifer and me. At weddings and parties we always go and claim an unoccupied corner – out of everyone's way – and "dance."

This dancing involves Jennifer elevating her powerchair seat so we're closer to the same height, and we either embrace and sway to a slow song or join hands and boogie with our arms to a fast song.

But there was something different this time at WCMU's annual Night of Louisiana.

This was our second year attending what the public broadcasting network flaunts as a way for people to cure the mid-winter blues. As for me, I always tell others they ***have*** to go because it's just plain ridiculous fun!

So, Jennifer and I donned our Mardi Gras beads and headed out for a night of southern-style cuisine and live Cajun and zydeco music by The Pine Leaf Boys and Lil' Nathan and the Zydeco Big Timers.

After meeting up with our friends, we swiftly forgot about the frigid late January freeze. Trusting in the sweet fruitiness of overpriced and fully liquored Hurricane drinks to cool the burn from our spicy Cajun dinner, Jennifer and I watched as people swarmed the dance floor three notes into The Pine Leaf Boys' opening song.

The people's dancing to the fiddle- and accordion-laced Cajun music was contagious. Jennifer and I quickly claimed a vacant

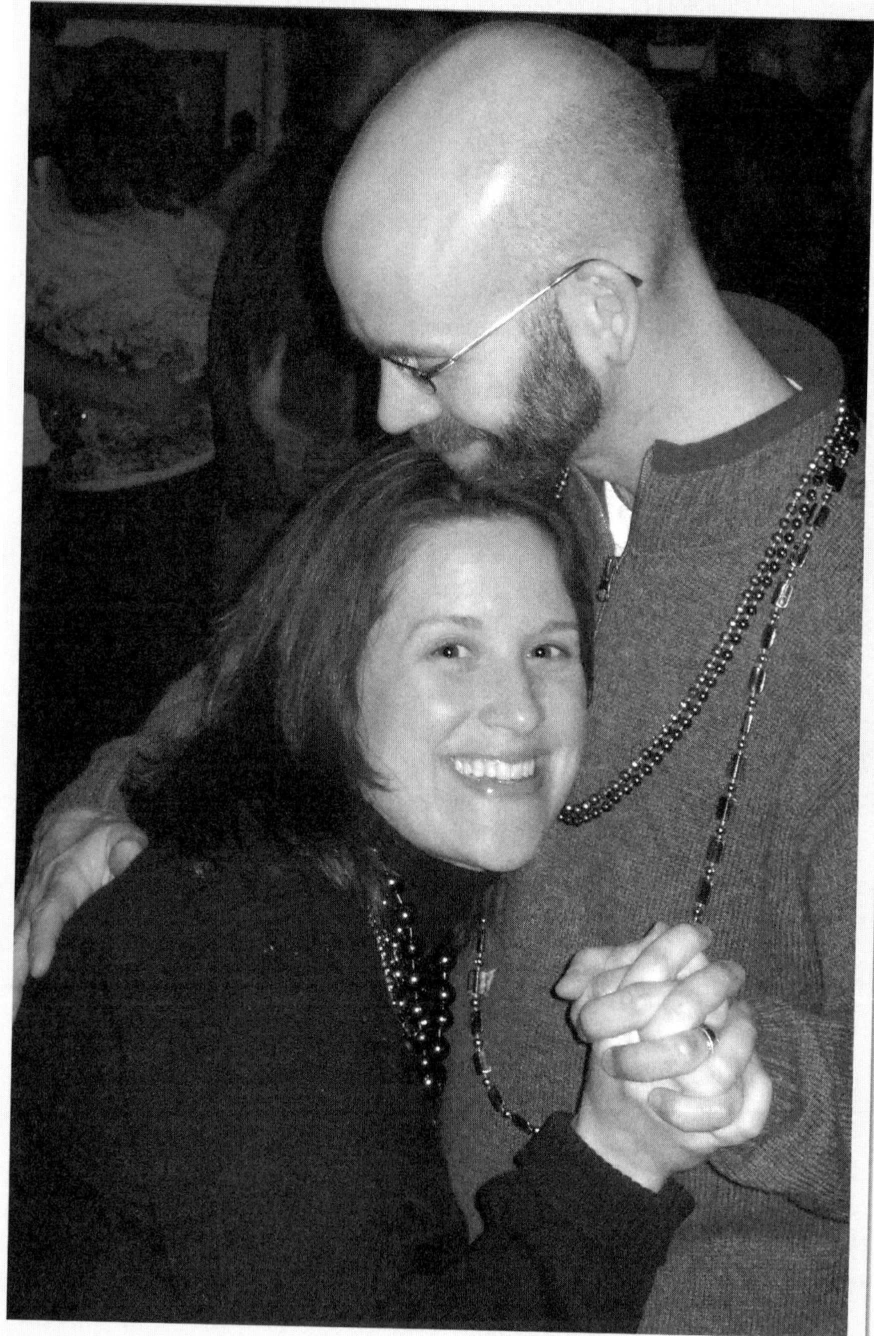

space on the dance floor and throughout the night we danced – swaying and boogying while Jennifer sat in her powerchair.

But with one song, everything changed: Jennifer was standing – honest to God standing! – with me out on the dance floor.

Lord knows what led us to give this a try (Jennifer thinks maybe it was a little liquid courage), but all I remember was her looking up at me as the slow song started and I asked, "Did you want to try standing a little for this one?"

Certainly, I always help Jennifer stand to make transfers at home, but never had we stood together like this in public, especially on a dance floor with hundreds of people around us.

Jennifer didn't hesitate to say, "Yes," and as we always do, she put her arms around my neck and I straddled her right leg, slightly squatted, wrapped my arms around her back and locked my hands together. And she counted, "1, 2, 3."

There we were. Dancing our first slow dance. Jennifer and I standing together swaying to the slow song. And all we really could do was smile as we looked into each other's eyes (although, I do remember telling her how awesome it was to see her standing because she knows how much I enjoy the fact that she's actually two inches taller than me).

While her MS-weakened legs likely limited our dance to less than a minute, I truly had lost track of time. I was *really* dancing with my wife. I'll bet as Jennifer stood with me, we looked just like everyone else on the dance floor.

But I couldn't tell you for sure. For that moment in time, we were the only ones out there.

Membership has its privileges

BY JENNIFER

Does "standing room only" apply to me anymore? After all, I no longer stand.

Yes, I'm being cheeky but something that happened earlier this week got Dan and me thinking.

Central Michigan University hosted many events to celebrate Martin Luther King Jr. Week, highlighted by a keynote performance by Danny Glover – yep, *Lethal Weapon* Danny Glover.

He, along with his lifelong friend Felix Justice, presented *An Evening with Martin & Langston.* This performance intended to "bring audiences inside the worlds of two of the greatest orators of the 20th century: Martin Luther King Jr. and Langston Hughes."

Sounds pretty interesting, right? It was a free performance with no tickets required. But, again, it was *Lethal Weapon* Danny Glover! How were Dan and I going to get accessible seats?

Dan knew I wanted to go so he called ahead, and they were able to accommodate us. And they weren't just any accessible seats: They were in the front row.

When we arrived 30 minutes before the performance, there was a line all the way down the hall with people trying to get seats in an already packed Plachta Auditorium. The ushers spotted us, called us forward and showed us to our seats right at the foot of the stage.

I was so excited and so appreciative that CMU made the performance accessible for me as well as two other people in wheelchairs. We ***were*** the front row. For *Lethal Weapon* Danny Glover!

As Dan and I turned around to see the mob of people lining the walls at the back of the auditorium, I leaned over and whispered to him, “Membership has its privileges.” It’s wrong to say, but I guess great seats are a perk of being disabled.

It was a powerful performance that we both enjoyed. When it was over, Dan leaned over to me and whispered, “Membership does have its privileges, but all things being equal, I would have given anything for you and me to be among those standing at the back of the auditorium for the entire performance because it would mean you didn’t have MS.”

And you know what? I would have too.

Laith Al-Saadi at the Gem

BY DAN

Jennifer and I are sitting here still reeling from less than four hours sleep last night. Perhaps it's a blues hangover or it's just our age telling us that we no longer can stay out late and get to bed after 2 a.m.

Either way, we did something last night that we've been talking about ever since we started listening to the Juke Joint with "The Duke of Juke" Robert Barclay on CMU Public Radio: We finally saw Ann Arbor-based rockin' blues man Laith Al-Saadi at The Gem Theater in St. Louis, Mich.

We first heard Laith's infectious groove, smooth vocals and powerful rock- and blues-driven guitar on the Juke Joint while we were stretching Jennifer's legs one Sunday evening. His song "Turn It Around" from his debut album, *Long Time Coming*, was like nothing we had ever heard before. We bought the disc and we've been hooked ever since.

Laith is a favorite of the blues crowd who frequent The Gem Theater, so he usually appears there several times each year. But, because it was a smaller venue, we figured it wasn't going to be handicapped accessible and didn't take the time to investigate whether Jennifer could get into the theater with her powerchair.

Too bad we didn't investigate sooner.

We were in the area and drove by The Gem to make sure it had no steps to enter the downtown building. After seeing the theater entrance was barrier free, we called about tickets.

We went into this figuring The Gem would not have a suitable accessible bathroom and, when Jennifer needed to use the restroom, we likely would have to leave early or go to the nearby McDonald's.

It was our lucky day because The Gem was first class. In fact, owner Minard Shattuck came up to us shortly after we arrived to let us know where the accessible restroom was located. Minard and his wife, Jenni, did everything they could to make this a comfortable and enjoyable experience for us.

And it was a great thing that the bathroom was perfect for us to use because Laith tore it up singing and jamming with his drummer and bass player for nearly four hours. That's right: FOUR HOURS!

We're already planning our next trip to The Gem Theater to enjoy another great blues show and have marked our calendar for the next time Laith will perform there.

A good pair of black pants

BY JENNIFER

Whether you are male or female, you probably have heard about the all-important "little black dress." Well for me, an outfit starts with "a good pair of black pants." You know those simple stylish pants that go with everything.

It has been a little over eight years since I've driven a car. Hate that, but I accept it. Been almost that long since I've walked. Yep, that stinks, but considering my disease, life could be much worse. Have to have help in the restroom. That one is hard to accept, but I do – begrudgingly. Again, it could be worse.

However, there is one thing in my life that MS affects that I no longer want to accept. It causes my almost daily complaints, and I hate to complain but here goes: I'm sick of Multiple Sclerosis' hold on my fashion.

Yes, my FASHION.

MS makes me question every clothing choice I make. That is so unfair. It's been at least seven years since I wore pants that button and zip. Yes, I hear some of you. Indeed, I know how a buttonhook works. But really, how practical is that?

And fun, flirty skirts. Well those just aren't practical for someone in a wheelchair. Or, honestly, very ladylike either. If I choose a longer skirt, it better cover my T.E.D. hose (my lovely white circulation, edema-alleviating stockings).

Speaking of T.E.D. hose, it's been years since I wore sandals. Not to brag but I do have cute toes. And shorts in the summer? Please! How silly would that be?

So when my wonderful friends and family invite me to social functions, my first thought is always, "What am I going to wear?"

And yes, I hear you Dad, my friends would still invite me if I wore a T-shirt and sweatpants, but is it too much to ask that I have fashionable, age-appropriate clothes?

I want to wear jeans. Real denim jeans – the kind with cute rinses and style. Not those made from light cotton fabric that only "look" like denim. They may work in the summer but come cold weather, what warmth is there in light cotton?

Don't get me wrong, I like and value my almost jeans. And I really appreciate pants with elastic waistbands, which simplify my dressing routine. But I long for buttons and zippers.

I've had plenty of events to get dressed up for this summer as invites to weddings, baby showers, super-nice National MS Society functions, and opportunities to share our story came my way.

But until fashion changes or until my disease miraculously goes away, you bet for most social occasions, I'll be wearing "a good pair of black pants."

What's a trip to Chicago without the Cubs?

BY JENNIFER

It was eight years ago today – September 28, 2010 – that I met Dan and told my mom, "He's really cute and sweet, but Mom, he likes Springsteen. Yuck! And he loves baseball. How boring!!"

Now eight years later, not only am I happily married to Dan, but I've seen Bruce in concert six times, loving every one of them. And on our honeymoon, we saw the Boston Red Sox play baseball in Toronto. So it shouldn't come as much of a surprise that we celebrated our fifth anniversary by meeting up with friends from Iowa to see a Cubs game in Chicago.

Dan and I, along with our friends Pam, Steve, D.J., and Deb found our seats in Wrigley field about 30 minutes before the first pitch.

Our seats were at the very back of the second tier on the third base side. And if you regularly read our blog or know my life with MS, you know a bathroom has to be part of this story. The family restrooms – the ones I use with Dan's help – unfortunately were located either on the level above or the level below us. Imagine having to wait for the elevator every time you had to go to the bathroom!

That's exactly what I had to do. But it only took me one such trip to the upperdeck before I got tired of making it. Luckily, we noticed vacant accessible seats closer to the family restroom, which coincidently had an incredible view of the ballpark. So I kindly asked a friendly usher, "How can we get seats like these? You know, ones closer to the bathrooms I use?" He understood my

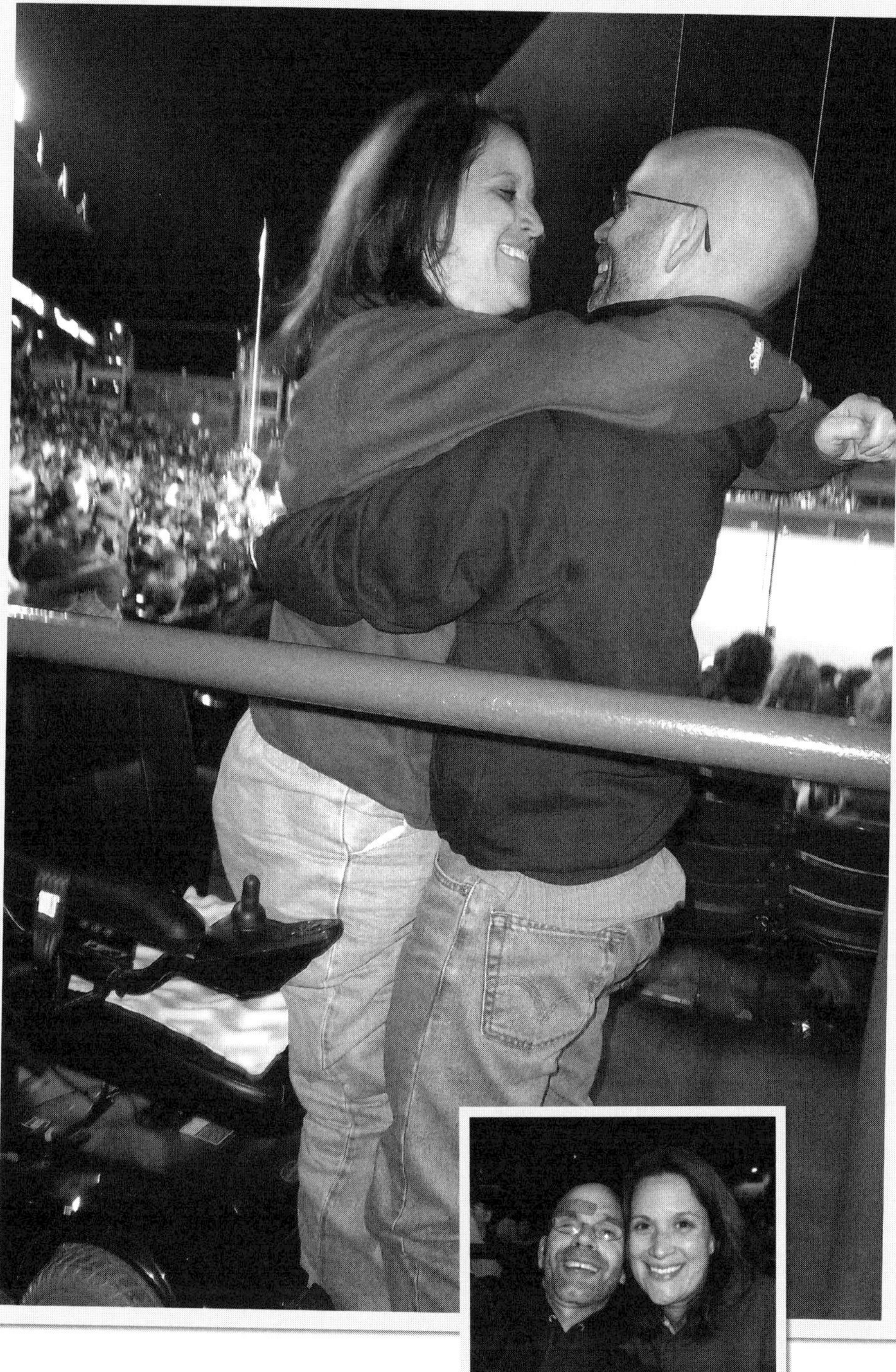

situation and encouraged me to check with Fan Services to inquire about upgrading our tickets.

Long story short: We were able to upgrade close to the family restroom on the first level, which landed us 10 rows from the field right behind home plate! It cost us a little more for these great seats, but it was SO worth it.

The night seemed to be perfect, but there had to be a way to get me and my powerchair that close to the field. This involved me taking a motorized chairlift. In helping to secure my chair to said chairlift, my loving husband stumbled – stupid numb MS feet – and he hit his head **hard**.

Dan had to be treated by the nurses in the ballpark's First Aid station. They were quick to treat him (no stitches needed) and he was back to the game before the second inning ended. Hence his name is forever on file at Wrigley Field ... granted it is in medical records but still, how many of us can say that?

The game was great, highlighted by standing with Dan during the seventh-inning stretch where Hall of Fame Chicago Bears running back Gale Sayers sang "Take Me Out to the Ball Game."

Speaking of singing, in the eighth inning three ballpark ushers sang "Happy Anniversary" to us and presented us with a ball used during the game. It even has dirt and scuffs on it. What a souvenir!

What a night for me, a girl who once hated baseball. A girl who doesn't let Multiple Sclerosis stand in the way of experiencing life. A great life with that cute man I met eight years ago.

3

It's Complex

A complex disease
and not just physically.
It tests emotions.

A common approach.
Most MSers employ it.
A good attitude.

Let's not feel guilty
if we slip and get depressed.
This is scary stuff.

–JUDY WILLIAMS

Guess what? MS doesn't cause all my health concerns

BY DAN

I was lying on my side watching the ultrasound monitor show my heart beating. I started laughing as I thought to myself, "Wow! That's my heart on that there Tee Vee!"

So, my heart is beating. That's good, Doc.

So, my existing minor heart condition – mitral valve prolapse – is confirmed. That's fine, Doc.

So, I have a slow heartbeat. That scares the hell outta me, Doc. What do you mean?

So, the normal range is 60 to 90 beats per minute and I checked in at 30 to 35. What can cause such a dreadful heartbeat, Doc? Tell it to me straight. I've been diagnosed with MS. I can handle it. And my lovely wife, Jennifer, I know she'll be strong enough for both of us. What did I do to deserve this?

So, yes I do exercise. I run about 40 minutes three or four days a week, Doc.

So, that explains, justifies and excuses my slow heartbeat, Doc. That's, good, I guess.

Seems like much of my health care is a guessing game.

Recurring lightheadedness is what led me to the doctor today. Every morning when I squat down to help Jennifer put on her socks and shoes, I get a rush of blood to my head when I stand up. The rush has been hitting me harder lately to the point I've had to pause several seconds to get my bearings and avoid passing out.

Turns out it has a lot of potential causes, including:

- **Mitral valve prolapse** – I've had this relatively minor (at least for me) heart condition that flares up only when I've had too much caffeine
- **Improper diet** – I'm a fully active person but sans breakfast I eat the same foods as Jennifer, who stringently adheres to her Weight Watchers diet to lose weight
- **Multiple Sclerosis** – That darn chronic disease of the central nervous system I've lived with for nearly 10 years.

Oftentimes people who have MS are quick to pinpoint the disease as the cause of every health concern. MS is powerful; I'll give him that. But I'd hate to think he'd get the best of me by taking all the credit for an entirely treatable symptom or condition that I missed fixing simply because I erroneously chalked it up to MS.

What I appreciate about my family physician is that he is willing to pause, assess the situation and make an educated medical guess, or hypothesis, if you will.

So, we started with the heart. I have one more heart exam tomorrow in Midland, and as luck would have it, my regular six-month check-up with my neurologist also is tomorrow in Midland.

Is my lightheadedness caused by my heart or my MS? Maybe one. Maybe the other. Maybe both. Maybe neither.

But I have a qualified physician and neurologist on my side. And their educated ~~guesses~~ hypotheses are better than mine.

BTW: My heart was causing these concerns, and by eating a little more and not standing up so quickly, everything is under control. It had nothing to do with MS.

Tearful trash talking

BY DAN

The white spots show where MS has left its mark on my brain.

I've lived my life with MS as though we're in a competition together. I trash talk it every day. Gotta be tough, ya know? Not that this chronic disease of the central nervous system cares what I have to say. I won't hurt its feelings. But I talk tough so it won't hurt mine.

Still, no matter how tough I talk after I throw down and capitalize on accomplishing another goal – everything from getting out of bed in the morning to finishing another training run or an organized race – I know this disease will bring me to tears at least once every other year.

I cried earlier this week.

My neurologist likes to do an MRI of my brain every other year to monitor the progression of the disease.

It's one of those things where even though I'm not experiencing any negative effects of MS on the surface, it doesn't mean MS isn't wreaking havoc throughout my central nervous system. The MRI is proof positive whether or not the disease has stealthily destroyed unused portions of my brain as I've naively gone about my business thinking I've kept this beast at bay.

I'm not going to lie: I peeked at the MRI scans before I took them into my neurologist. Not that I could tell what any of them specifically meant, but I know enough to look for the white spots on the brain. These spots are the scarring, or sclerosis – evidence

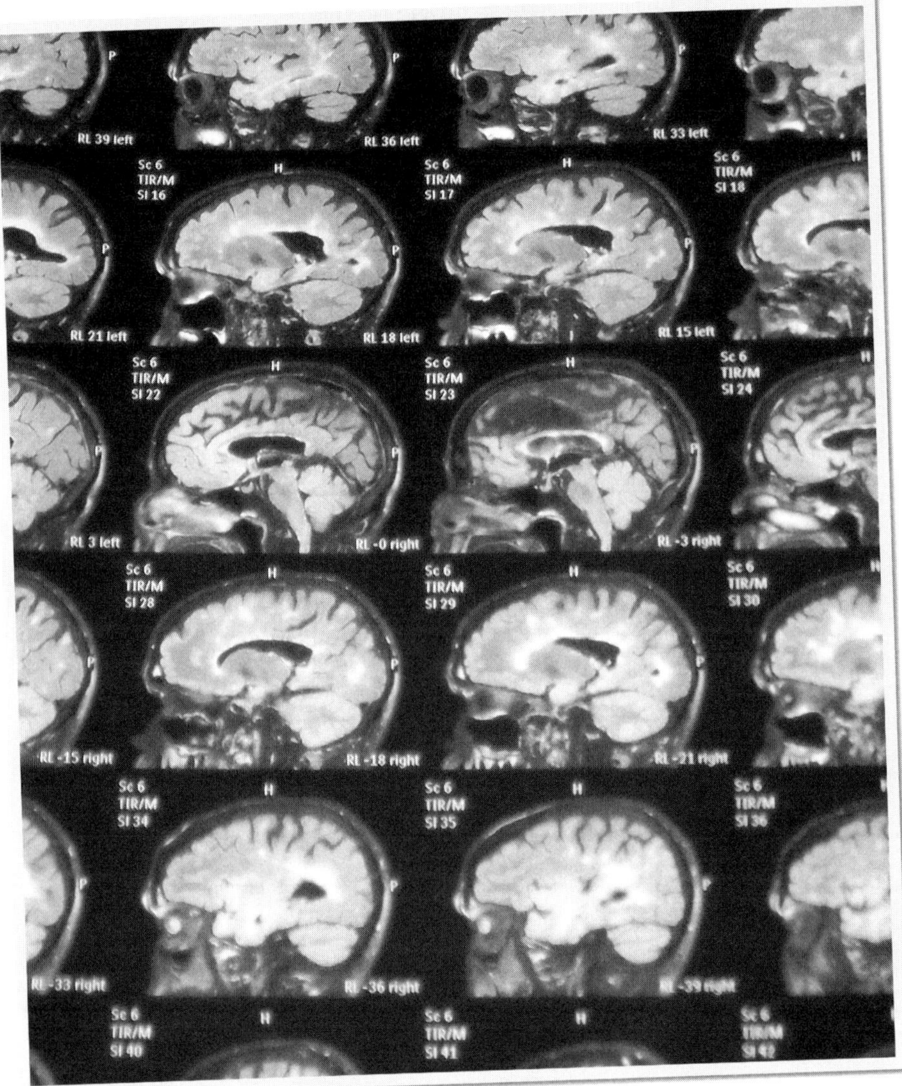

of where my immune system has mistakenly attacked the myelin sheath surrounding my nerve cells.

As always, I got a little short of breath when I knew I found the scan I was looking for. I wondered to myself whether there were too many white spots this time. Is this worse than it was before? Or is it the same? Maybe it's worse. Wait. Don't read into it,

Dummy. It's probably nothing. But how can I tell? I can't. And I won't.

So I prayed. Not that I prayed it wouldn't be bad news, but for the strength to handle whatever news I received. Interesting thing to note is that you can connect with God even if you don't fold your hands. God is good that way. I mean, come on. It's God.

Like a criminal awaiting his sentencing, I stood firm when my neurologist clipped THE scan to the light board in the exam room. Pointing to the scan that I had feared, he said something to the effect that this one looked just like it did two years ago, and he confirmed what the radiologist had reported each time I've had an MRI over the past decade.

"There is no progression in the disease. Everything is stable."

And as I always have done following each MRI for the past decade, I saved my tears for the car.

Then I trash talked the disease all the way home.

Am I really disabled?

BY JENNIFER

Sounds like such a stupid question. Me, the one living with Multiple Sclerosis for the last nearly 13 years, but almost every morning I wake up thinking, "Just give me a second. I'll jump out of bed and get moving." Silly right? But, my dreams play a small part in this deluded thought. Stupid dreams! I still walk in them, how deceptive and unfair is that?

Since I met Dan, I have never walked. But in my dreams, we often walk together into crazy, nonsensical adventures all of the time – hey, dreams don't have to (and trust me mine don't) make sense. I guess it's good that I still walk in them because it reminds me what I'm fighting for. I believe, I HAVE to believe, I will walk again.

But am I really disabled?

You'd think, the wheelchair or the reality I can no longer roll over in bed or get to the toilet without help might tell me I am. But, un-uh. Still don't see myself that way. As for those little blue wheelchair signs designating handicapped parking spots and restrooms, those are just signs. That's not me!

This lack of acceptance, i.e. denial, might explain my constant frustration and frequent tearful outbursts when no one is looking. But those are mine to live and deal with, and pity is certainly not acceptable or being asked for.

But again I ask, am I really disabled?

Recently, I was asked by the office of Student Disability Services to tell the Facilities Management staff at Central

Michigan University how they could improve the handicap accessibility of their buildings. Guess that should've been a clue, but truly, it was the two women in wheelchairs I met that night that made me doubt the genuineness of my disability.

They also were providing the FM staff valuable feedback on building improvements. Only they were sharing stories of cruising their power chairs around campus, or through town, the daily difficulties of riding public transportation, or having to replace worn out wheels.

I couldn't relate. After all, I ride in my van and can't imagine driving my chair enough to wear out my wheels' tread. Really, I'm only kind of disabled.

But when they started talking about getting stuck in the snow or having slippery wheels from said snow and about hard-to-open power assist doors, I started to relate.

Then the topic turned to the best handicapped restrooms on campus. And when we all knowingly exclaimed, "Park Library. Definitely the library," it started to sink in. I was with my peers.

Sure my MS support group is full of people who understand this disease, but none of our regulars use a wheelchair. And Dan, he provides tremendous support and understanding. But it was in that room with those women in wheelchairs that it began to be OK.

Yes, I really am disabled. And after not walking for the past eight years, you are probably thinking, "Well duh! Finally." But for the first time, I felt comfortable enough to say, "I am disabled." (Of course with the caveat, "I make disabled look good!")

And maybe now, I'll even be OK with photos of me in my chair. Um. OK, probably not. Call me vain, but I'm thinking I'll still crop it out.

Becoming the bat man

BY DAN

It began in mid-October when my hands, chest and feet started feeling numb. The numbness, of course, was my penance for being a weekend athlete and stretching my body to the point that I had pinched a nerve. I needed to have my doctor take a look.

I came home from work to put on jeans and the Bruce Springsteen T-shirt I had bought at a concert the month earlier. After partially covering Springsteen with a red flannel shirt, I got my tennis shoes from the entryway and headed to the doctor's office.

Sitting in the exam room, I felt some crowding in my right shoe. I concluded that I hadn't put on my sock correctly and it had folded under my foot. I leaned over and removed my shoe. Then I heard an agitated kind of chirping sound from deep inside my size 8-1/2 crosstrainer.

Funny, I thought, I don't remember seeing crickets in the entryway.

I only wish I had found a cricket.

There was a bat in my shoe. A nocturnal flying mammal with membranous wings. A BEADY-EYED BAT IN MY SHOE!

How could I keep it contained? I ripped off my flannel shirt and covered my shoe. I then scurried outdoors to free the bat.

I feared it would fly up into my face if I merely tapped my shoe on the parking lot curb. I figured it would be best to spike my shoe onto the pavement like a football player after scoring a touchdown.

Four times I slammed my footwear to the ground. On my fifth attempt, the bat tumbled onto the curbside. It was limp, almost lifeless. I'm sure it had one heck of a headache.

Carrying my shoe and flannel shirt, I retreated to the exam room. The doctor entered a few minutes later.

"How are you doing today?" he asked.

"I have to tell you something," I said with a twinge of panic in my voice. "This is sooooo not related to why I'm here, but ..." and I told him everything.

"There was a bat," he clarified.

Yes.

"And it was in your shoe?"

Yes.

He asked whether the bat had bitten me. Not that I knew of, but then again, my feet were numb. He checked my foot and called his nurse to have her report the incident to the health department.

He also wanted me to have some blood drawn for testing. As he concluded the exam, the nurse knocked on the door.

"The health department would like to talk with Dan," she said.

I got on the phone with the health department nurse, and I told her everything.

"There was a bat?"

Yes.

"And it was in your shoe?"

Yes.

"Is it still alive?" she asked.

I don't know.

"We need you to go out and see if it's still there, and call us back."

The bat barely had moved from the curbside.

"Still there," I said in my return call.

"Well, we need you to try and catch it," she said.

And I need you to try and get real, I thought.

"I'll do what I can," I said.

"If you catch it, we need you to bring it here so we can test it for rabies."

I invoked my MacGyver-like instincts and corralled the bat using a plastic container and a piece of cardboard. I placed the container in my car, and went inside to have my blood drawn.

From down the hall the laboratory technician walked toward me shouting, "Ya lookin' for a vampire?"

What?! Does news here travel that fast?

Turns out her question was just lab tech humor. She had no idea what had happened, so I told her everything.

I then drove to the health department and turned in my bat. The woman instructed me to call the next day for the test results. I guess I figured I'd be all right as long as I didn't start foaming at the mouth.

Turns out the bat wasn't rabid. But the medicine my doctor prescribed didn't cure the numbness, and, after undergoing numerous tests, I was diagnosed with Multiple Sclerosis. Some pinched nerve.

Because of the medicine I'm taking to slow the disease's progression, I have to go in every three months for a blood test.

The lab technician knows my name, but she still gets a kick out of calling me "the bat man."

This article originally appeared in the membership magazine of the National MS Society (Inside MS).

MS at 2 a.m. in an Orlando E.R.

BY JENNIFER

It's been a little more than six months since Dan's and my trip to Walt Disney World. My memories from that, um, memorable trip are still pretty fresh.

Let's see, I remember theme park rides, amazing fireworks, images of Mickey Mouse everywhere and having a great time with my family and Dan. But really what I remember most is my late-night visit to Celebration Hospital in Orlando.

To treat my MS, I take a subcutaneous injection every day, which is supposed to lessen the frequency and severity of my Multiple Sclerosis. After giving myself daily injections for the last 12 years, I guess it was bound to happen: I had to have an incident to remember.

And remember this one I will.

It was a little later than when I usually take my shot, but we were on vacation – getting away from it all. The day was pretty packed with activities. Eating dinner, taking my shot, and crawling into bed sounded like a perfect ending to a busy Disney day.

I took my pre-filled syringe from the refrigerator, pulled off the cap, inserted the needle into my stomach, and pushed on the plunger. But the plunger didn't budge. This sometimes is typical because I've developed scar tissue from taking so many injections. As usual, I asked Dan to push in the fluid. He pushed on the plunger, but it still didn't move.

I gave it another try and in my brilliance, I thought, "Oh, just give it a little twist." And the next thing I knew, I had a syringe in one hand, and a needle in my stomach. Understandably, I started to freak out. But I tried to stay calm, looking at Dan to fix it. I was pleading with my eyes, "Fix this," and he was looking at me with confused, "I wish I could" eyes.

Just then, he took his fingers and tried to grab the pointed metal piece and well, you know how quicksand in movies looks? That's how the needle disappeared into my belly.

Poof. It was gone.

"Oh no! Oh no! What am I going to do?" I frantically questioned.

Dan was as mystified as I was. What could we do? I tried to regain some calm and call the hotel front desk.

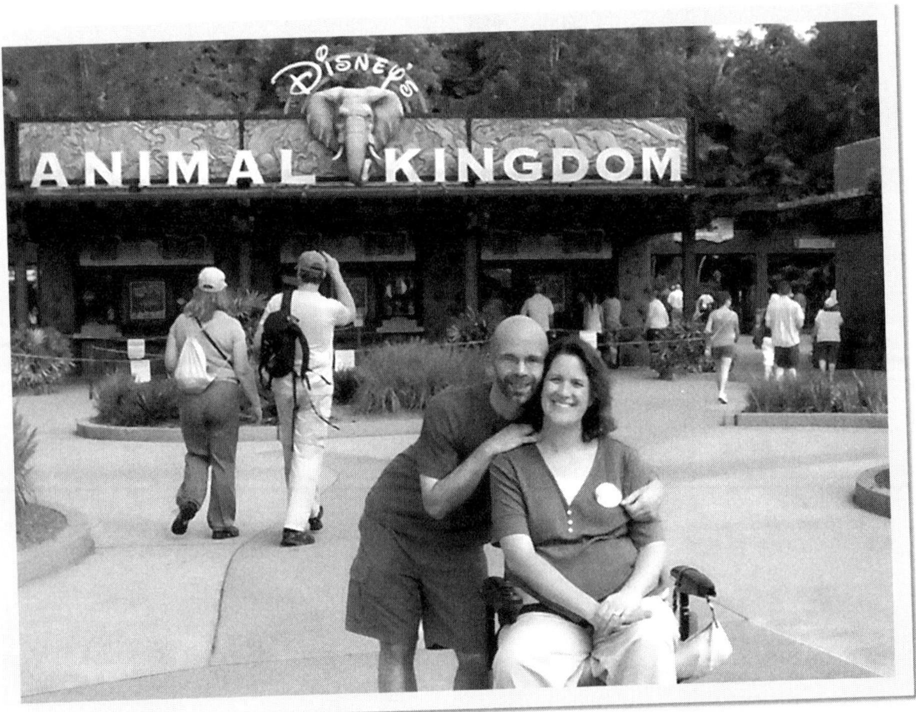

They transferred me to hotel safety, where I gave the same story I just told you. Safety was as mystified. They told me to call paramedics, which I did. When they arrived I went through the whole story again and they said, "We've never heard of that. You should probably go to the hospital and at least have an X-ray."

So off to the hospital we went. X-rays were taken. At least three times – between doctors and nurses and X-ray techs – I heard, "Wow, never heard of that before." Comforting, isn't it? By about 2 a.m., after several X-rays turned up nothing, the doctor told me that he was going to let the needle work itself out, kind of like a sliver. After all, it would be more dangerous to perform surgery to remove something they couldn't see.

Guess what I said? "Really, hmm, I've never heard of that before." But I trusted him, and besides, I just wanted to go home; home to Michigan, that is.

Because the reality is, when you live with a chronic illness like MS, you never really can get away from it all.

BTW: It really turned out to be a great trip – and as of June 2011, the souvenir needle still is somewhere in my belly.

The fine art of shooting myself

BY DAN

It seems like years ago that I anxiously investigated how to go about shooting myself.

The information was all right there in front of me. Books. Brochures. Videos. Each included a map of the human body that highlighted the areas where it would be most effective to do the shooting.

Empty silhouettes of the body that had betrayed each of us with MS, who now are made to sit there reading said books and brochures and watching the aforementioned videos that were saturated with forced optimism to put us at ease.

It will be easy to do, they all said. Here: Take a nice plump orange and practice the proper procedure. An apple would do but an orange better simulates the density of human flesh. Soft, human flesh. Packaged neatly in a fragrant ball stamped "Sunkist."

After several botched attempts, I think I finally got the hang of it. I discover that the key to the proper technique of shooting myself: "It's all in the wrist."

Just like others had told me to do, I have the bottle of ibuprofen on the table next to my supplies. It'll help with the pain. But take it at least 30 minutes before. It's pointless to plan on taking it after I shoot myself. It won't do much good.

Shut up and do it already, Dan.

Now a decade later, I'll take two ibuprofen and break open the supplies Jennifer lovingly has set out for me. Interesting how I'll

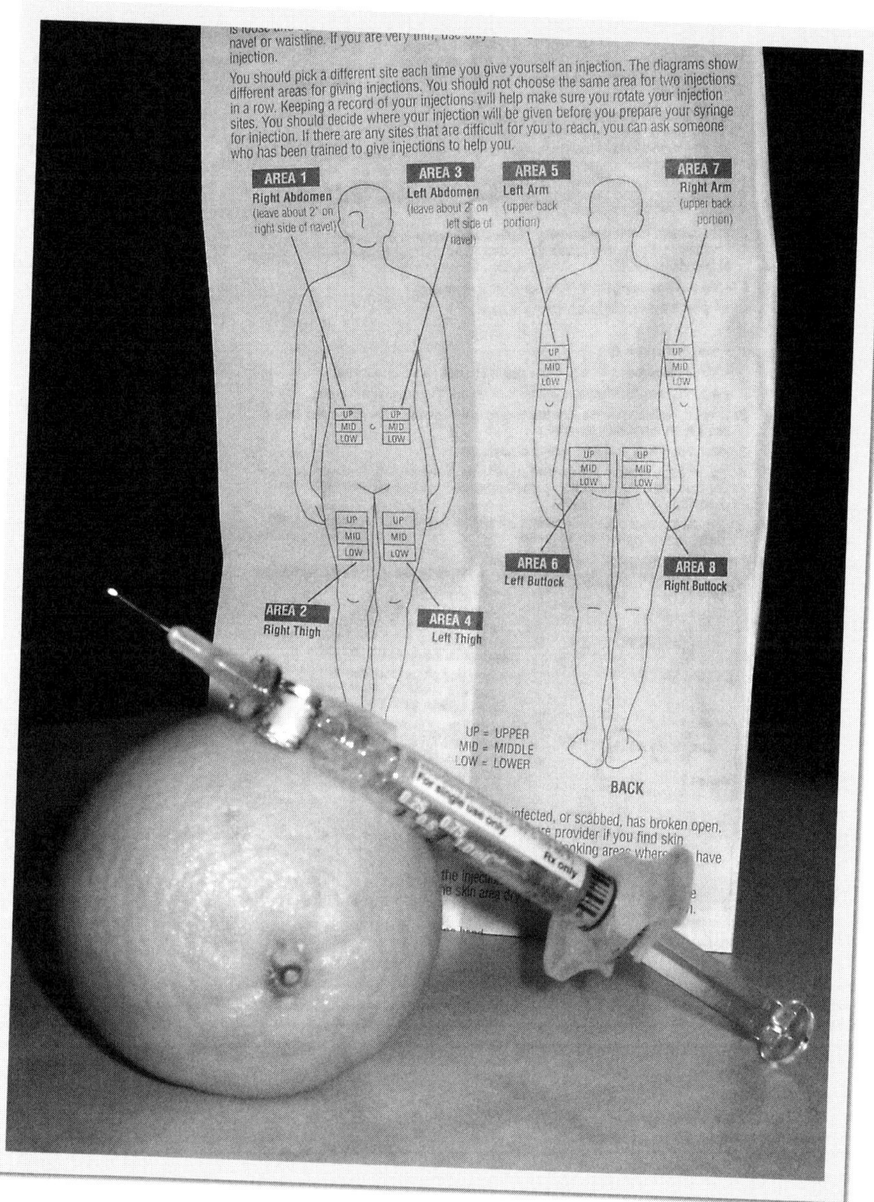

take two generic ibuprofen to alleviate the pain of a medicine that is produced and manufactured by the folks at Bayer.

Everything is neatly enclosed in a self-contained plastic package, plastic with the exception of the paper backing that I easily tear off to unleash the contents.

I first grab the vial containing the white powder that looks like what Hollywood says is cocaine. This white powder is what they say is the medicine that will help to slow the progression of my Multiple Sclerosis. Pop off the cap and strategically position it in the mixing spot reserved for it in the self-contained plastic package that by some stroke of engineering genius serves as both a container and medicine mixing station. An alcohol swab is placed on top briefly to fight off contamination.

I push the vial adapter, complete with a subcutaneous needle, onto my medicine mix, twist the stopper off the prefilled saline syringe that then is twisted onto the vial adapter. Again. A stroke of engineering genius.

Positioning the newly assembled engineered apparatus at a 45-degree angle, I slowly push the syringe to release the saline into the medicine vial. The angle is key because, much like a bartender carefully pours a beer into a glass from the side to limit the size of the head, or "footch" as my dad calls it, the liquid needs to flow into the vial the same way as to avoid making bubbles.

I mix the medicine in a slow swirling, not shaking, motion. Again. The bubbles.

Guided by the same measures that determine when gelatin is completely dissolved, I determine all is ready.

Tonight I'll shoot one of three specified regions on my left leg. I hate shooting my belly, I just did my arm last night, and I'll save my hip for another time. A second alcohol swab sanitizes my skin, and BAM! I give myself a shot.

But there's no bartender. No gun. Just me, my medicine, and my MS. And a life that is so worth living because of it.

The best medicine

BY JENNIFER

Fun … that's it. Really! Having a good time makes my MS more tolerable, and when I'm having lots and lots of fun, I sometimes even forget that I'm living with this disease. It's the good times and the people that I'm enjoying them with that motivate me to wake up every morning and keep fighting; and thus fun is *the best medicine!*

So without further ado, here is a glimpse at what has kept me (and Dan) busy:

Hey Boo-Boo

We went to a great picnic, and there is nothing better than being surrounded by friends who *just get you*. Friends from my old MS support group in Flint were getting together. A picnic was planned, but Dan and my attendance was spontaneous. Talking with two of the group's members earlier that afternoon, they mentioned their plans and invited us to join them at that evening's picnic. There was no way we would miss it! And even though I have not been to that group in the four years since I got married, I wanted to enjoy a nice summer evening with them and my husband. This event was so awesome because even though it was the disease that brought us together, it was barely mentioned. This picnic was about good food, good friends and good, oops I mean GREAT, times.

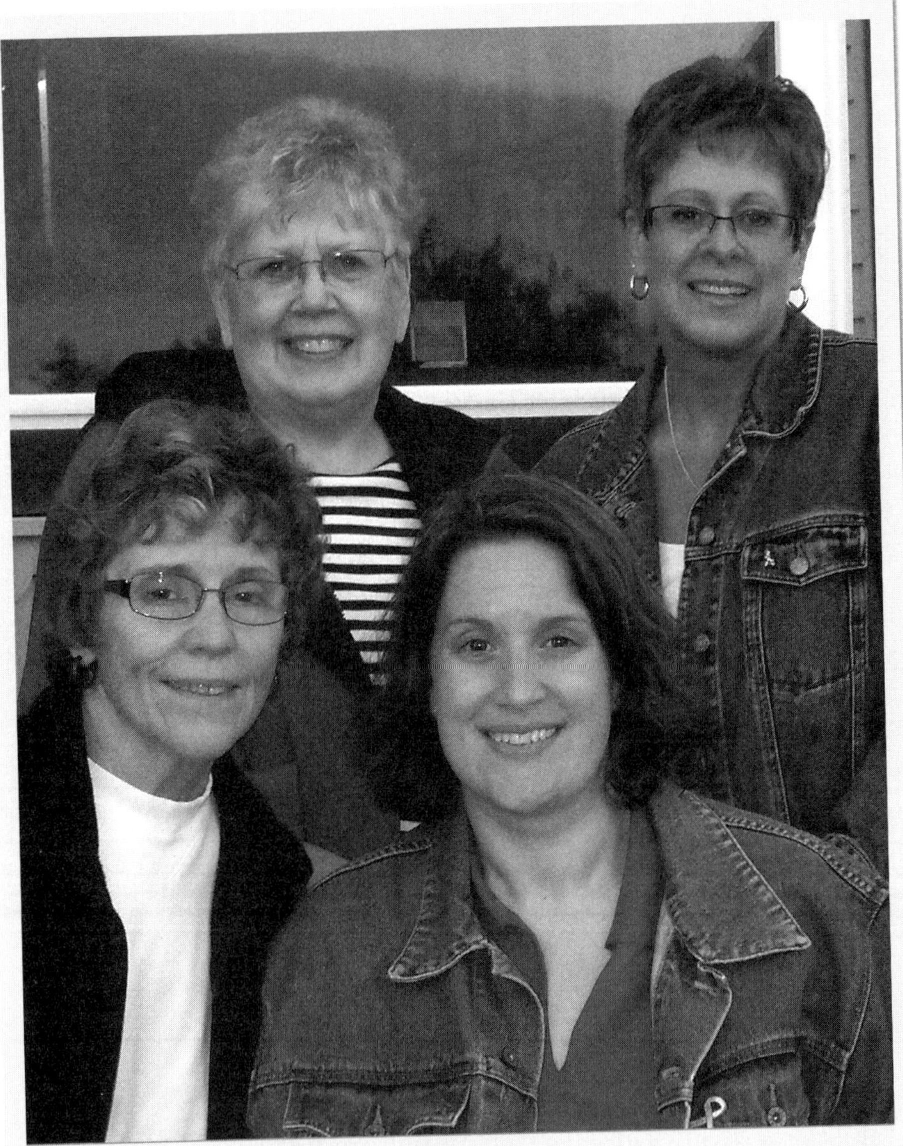

Play ball!

No not me, silly. *Watch* ball is more accurate. Dan, my dad, and Jim (my caregiver) and his family, and I went for a fun time at Dow Diamond in Midland. We saw a Great Lakes Loons baseball game. The Loons won! We ate too much – hot dogs, nachos, cotton candy, and of course, for me the required dill pickle – you know, the usual baseball essentials. Bonus, the weather provided us with a beautiful night! The recently built stadium is completely handicapped accessible, right down to a family restroom. This essential accommodation makes my comfort and enjoyment an almost certainty. And the cherry on top of this all-American sundae? After trying at the last few games we attended, I finally got to meet the team mascot, Lou E. Loon. What a perfect, fun evening!

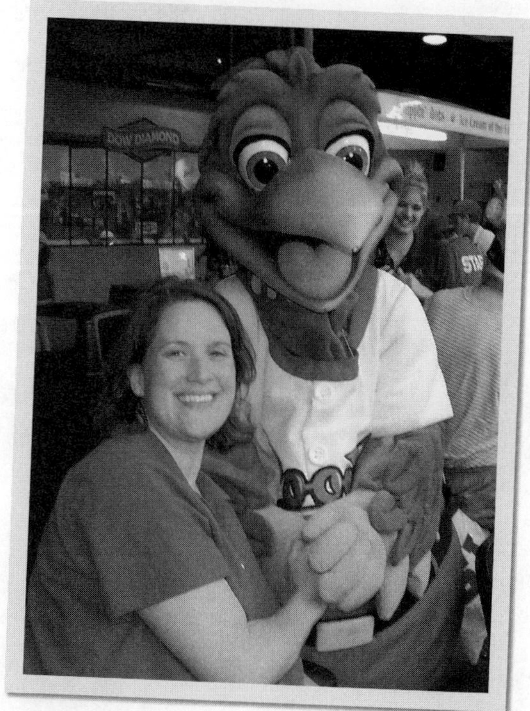

A man on a mission

After joining our team at this year's Walk MS a few months ago, Jake (the wonderful husband of my close college friend Heather) decided that I was going to be able to get into their house. See, we had been to their house last summer for a party following the Crim race in Flint, but I couldn't get into their house because it had a series of steps.

Jake wanted to ensure that I could see the inside of their house when he and Heather hosted the engagement party for our dear friends, Jen and Adam. So he did some research to see what was

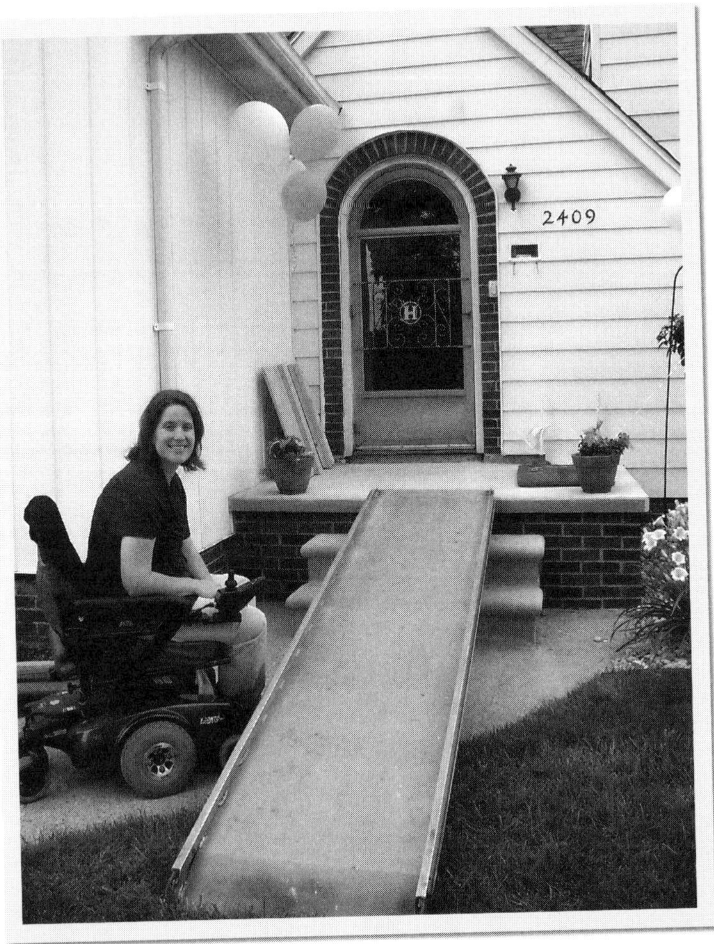

available. And, after asking me the width of my power wheelchair, he was fairly confident that he had found a solution: His friend Andy had access to a ramp from a standard moving truck. That, along with a custom ramp Jake built, made it possible for me to get into their house, which was very lovely, by the way. Once in their home I was able to use its bathroom, making it the first residential bathroom – other than ours and my parents' – that I've been able to use since I lost the ability to walk. Because of this, we could stay at the party for as long as we (and for a change not my bladder) wanted. And much fun was had! Thanks again, Jake and Andy.

Dan and I deal with MS every second of our lives, so isn't it great when we can find fun escapes? We're excited about the St. Louis Blues Festival over the Fourth of July, going to another Loons game, the annual Mount Pleasant MS group pizza party, another Crim race and post-race soiree, and whatever fun opportunities come our way.

Is it possible to have too much fun? Maybe, but we'll keep having as much as we can handle.

Now go have a little fun of your own!!

What would you do?

BY DAN

In a surreal sort of way, I felt like the bad guy in a situation stripped straight from ABC's hidden camera ethical dilemma series, *What Would You Do?* hosted by John Quinones.

But I had every reason and right to have our van parked in a handicapped parking spot close to Anspach Hall even after I just finished running my four-mile route on Central Michigan University's Mount Pleasant campus.

Part of me felt guilty, the other part was just itching for somebody to call me out on it. Unfortunately, nobody ever did.

But had someone ever asked how I – a runner – could get away parking in a handicapped spot, here is what I was ready to tell this bold person:

Thank you so much, and it's interesting you should ask me. I appreciate your concern. You see, my wife is disabled and I park here for her. She's in class right now, and each week I come up here so I can help her use the restroom during her break. After I help her, I go for a run.

I usually finish running about the same time her three-hour class is dismissed. I go up to get her on the second floor and carry her books – I'm chivalrous like that – and we take the elevator down and she drives her power wheelchair into our van parked here in this handicapped accessible spot.

Why is she disabled? No, that's not too personal of a question. She has Multiple Sclerosis. It's the secondary progressive kind of this chronic illness of the central nervous system. She no longer can walk. It's unpredictable and affects everyone differently. You see, I – the runner –

also have Multiple Sclerosis. Mine is the relapsing remitting kind. Did you see how I was stumbling a little after I got done running? Right. It affects everyone differently.

Suppose that's why I was itching for someone to call me on it. Not that I wanted a confrontation. It just felt like an ideal teaching moment for a university campus.

So if you saw something like this, what would you do?

Grape Ape

BY JENNIFER

"Hmm, what's today's date?" he asks before writing on the huge stack of paperwork.

I answer that it is February 20.

"Not bad, let's see," he shuffles through the forms. "Ordered this on November 4. That means it's been a little more than three months. Really, not bad, huh?"

I answer him, "Nope, not bad at all." But all the while I'm thinking, "You weren't the one stuck sitting in a wheelchair, sitting on a painful pressure sore for the last six months (because actually, I'd been treating it that long – but hey, who's counting?)."

Honestly Roger – the salesman from Saginaw Medical – Karen and Sue – the wound care specialists who treated my sore – and my doctors and social workers did a great job filling out oodles of forms, dotting all the i's and crossing all the t's that were necessary to help me get my snazzy new power wheelchair.

My Grape Ape.

So named for its pretty purple base and because I was a kid in the '80s when the cartoon character Grape Ape was popular. By naming my chair, like every other one I've had, the chair becomes mine and a name makes it more real.

Yes, it's real. My chair. My MS. And hate it as I did, the real truth is that like it or not, I need this chair.

I hope that you have gathered from its name, it's a big, powerful chair. It's not small. Not subtle like my old chairs Fred and Belle were. No messing with this chair. It means business. It has hydraulics, a headrest, and better foot positioning to relieve pressure from sitting all day, every day.

I need a chair that relieves pressure and fortunately this one does. It's bigger but as strange as it sounds, its size makes me uncomfortable.

I'm uncomfortable because does this mean my MS is worse? Will it make people look at me differently? Do I care? Will Dan and my caregivers still be able to transfer me? Will I see myself differently?

Lots of questions. Not a lot of answers. That is so typical of this stupid disease.

But for right now, I'm just sitting comfortably. Kind of forgot how good that feels.

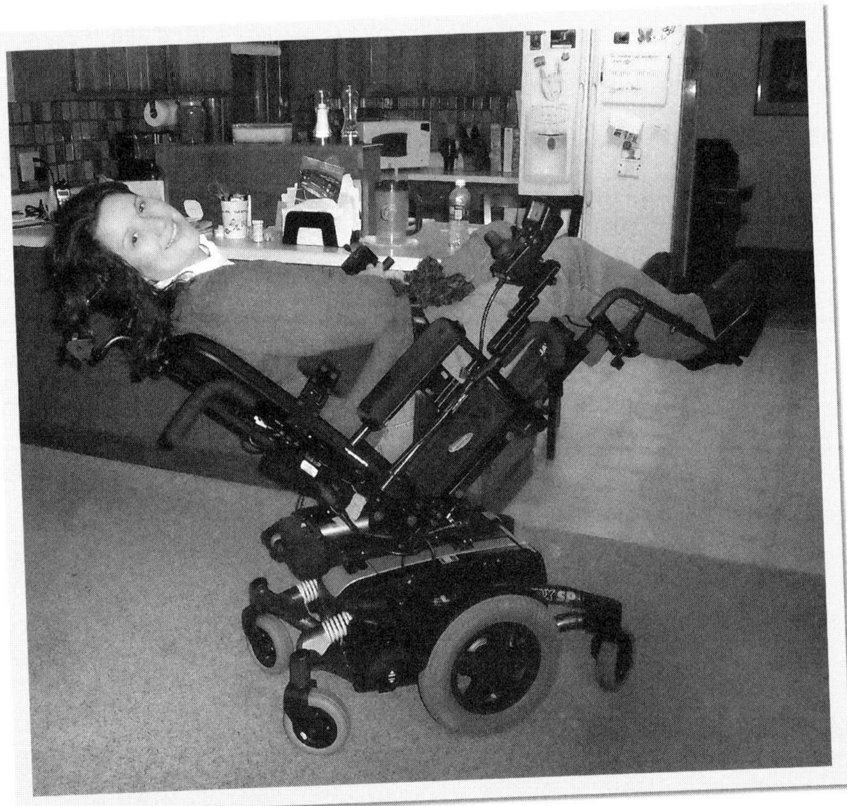

4

When One Finds Out . . .

The diagnosis,
its impact is life changing
hard to minimize.

There will remain things
one can control for the good.
Best to focus there.

Diet, exercise,
emotions, and attitude.
Those one can direct.

– JUDY WILLIAMS

Jennifer was right

BY DAN

Between a wall showcasing every major brand of running shoe in stock and a wall displaying the industry's best wicking apparel, the helpful salesman at Runners in Mount Pleasant squats and watches my feet as I walk back and forth on the uncarpeted section of the floor.

His analysis of my gait determines that I'm a neutral, meaning my foot absorbs the shock the way it was designed to, as opposed to landing heel or on the very outside of the foot first. He tells me what type of shoe I need.

He smirks when I ask him to settle an ongoing debate between Jennifer and me about my status of "being a runner."

Jennifer wholeheartedly professed that I was a runner, citing that I live and die by my Garmin GPS-enabled sports watch results each time I run and that I have respectable finishes in every race I enter. I, in turn, stressed that I wasn't a runner. I merely was a guy who runs, pointing out that I maintained nowhere near the gazelle-like physique and pace of the people I pictured as true runners.

"You know what the difference is between a jogger and a runner?" he asks.

"An entry form," he explains with a smile.

Following his logic, I'll agree with Jennifer's claim that I am a runner. But my numb feet always remind me that I am a runner who has MS.

Most races break down their entrants by specific age groups, not by whether or not they have MS. But if they did, I potentially have finished in the top five of this specific category in every race I've ever entered. Race forms will never single out runners who have MS, so I'll continue comparing myself to other runners who likely aren't living with this chronic disease.

I may never win any of the races I enter, but I always will have a decent showing because I'm there.

To spite my MS.

Fearlessness lost … and found

BY DAN

As much as I hate to admit it, Multiple Sclerosis had me running scared.

In the weeks leading up to the Alma Highland Festival held over Memorial Day weekend I was soooo afraid of falling. I guess the "Friday Night Incident on Mission Street" in late March had cut me deeper than the incident-instigated five-stitch gash on my forehead.

On that infamous Friday night, it was just supposed to be an easy training run. Nice weather. New running shoes. Bruce Springsteen's recent release on my iPod. A different route celebrating spring's return.

Less than two miles into my run I ventured beyond the friendly confines of the Central Michigan University campus and onto the sidewalks and parking lots along Mount Pleasant's busy Mission Street. Trucks and cars congested the street's four lanes. People on their way home from work. Families on their way to dinner. Friends on their way out for the night.

I still hope nobody saw me as I ran past Sherwin Williams in the strip mall across from Walgreen's. My left foot clipped the crack where the parking lot met the sidewalk.

It's bizarre to say it happened so quickly I had no time to react, yet at the same time I remember thinking countless thoughts during this split second, "You gotta be kidding me. I clipped the sidewalk and I'm gonna fall. I sure hope this doesn't hurt. Man, there's a lot of traffic and how graceful do I look? Don't flail, Dan. Fall. But for God's sake don't flail. It'll look so uncool."

BAM! My head, throttled by the momentum of my modest pace, smacked onto the pavement. Truly face first. Lying prostrate on the cold concrete I remember staring at a loose stone as the sting from the fall set into my skin and consciousness. I then shot up as quickly as I fell. "Nothing to see here, folks. I'm OK," I thought, as dime-sized drops of blood splashed onto the sidewalk and my new shoes. I turned off my iPod. Not now, Bruce. I think I hurt myself.

It's as though my forehead, left shoulder and left pinky had broken my fall and protected my legs, which was good because it ended up being a really long walk home. I'm grateful I was wearing a long-sleeved red shirt that night to camouflage the crimson mess I continually wiped off my forehead.

One college student stopped me to see if I was OK. "Does it look as bad as I think it does?" I asked him as he offered to call me a cab to get me home and to the emergency room. I appreciated his offer, but all I wanted was to get home to Jennifer. She'd make everything better.

Finally. Home. Jennifer all but started crying at the shock of it all. So did I. We spent nearly four hours at the E.R., where medical professionals stitched my head, wrapped my knuckles and X-rayed my poor left pinky. They said it was fine, but I still think I broke it.

Certainly this wasn't the first time I had fallen while running, but it was the first time in a long time it had happened. Was it my MS? After all, because of MS, as I get tired my left side gets a little weaker and I start dragging my left foot. This is why the last thing Jennifer always tells me before I go running is, "Pick up your feet."

I was out running just three days after I fell. I seemed to be moving quite well. That is, until I entered my first 5K race of the season. It was hosted by the CMU Physical Therapy Student Organization and coincidentally benefitted the National MS Society. I fell in the middle of the race. Again, my left foot clipped a raised crack in the sidewalk. Even though I scuffed my knuckles in the fall, I protected my head and finished the race in an OK time.

Two falls in less than a month. Was my MS getting worse? Was it time to back off on running?

At the end of the race Jennifer glared at my scuffed knuckles and declared, "'You need to get rid of those shoes. I'm going to buy

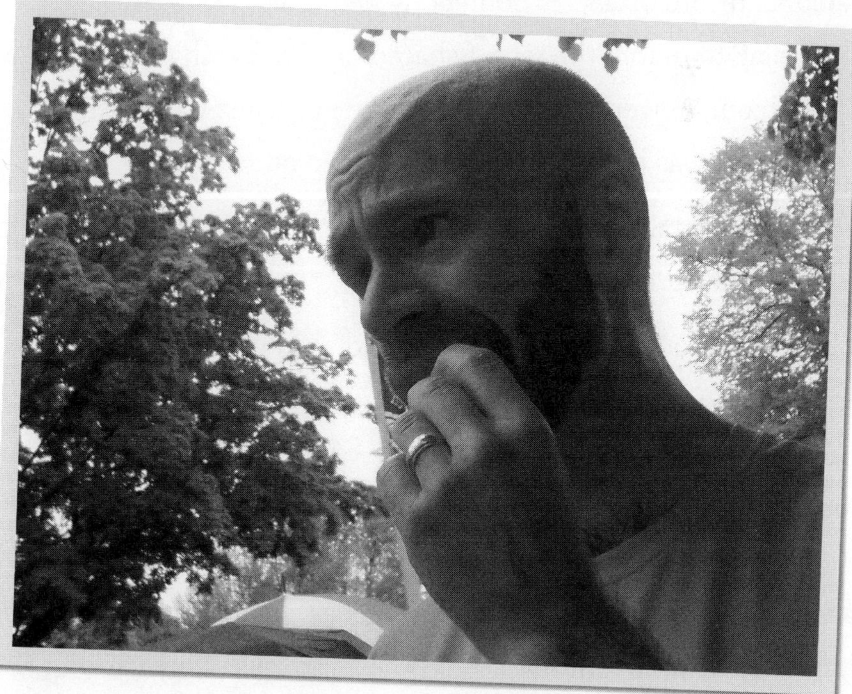

you some different ones this afternoon. It's not the MS. It's those damn shoes!" Excellent point, Detective Digmann. In the six times I had worn those new shoes, this marked the second time that I had fallen. So we went to Runners and bought some new shoes.

And while I hoped the newer new shoes would be my saving grace, my fear of falling had me running scared. Case in point: Two weeks later in my second 5K of the season – Central Michigan Community Hospital's Run-a-Trail – I finished in 26:44, more than two minutes slower than my 24:06 mark in the same race just a year ago.

I just couldn't shake the fear. Training runs. Running hills. Speed training. I didn't want to fall. But I was starting to feel some pressure. The Highland Festival was a mere three weeks away and it was at the festival's 5K race last year that I ran my overall personal record of 23:19. Somebody help me!

The night before the race, I shared my fears with Jennifer. And through our conversation she helped me to realize three things:

- The first was that I had every reason to be scared
- The second was that if I held back in my running so I wouldn't fall, that's precisely why I would fall

So I went out the next morning and I ran hard, never once thinking about falling despite the steady rain and wet course. I finished in 24:41; placing seventh out of 15 in my age group. I needed that.

Oh yeah, and the third thing I realized the night before the race? I needed to remember and embrace the Japanese proverb that had helped me through the earliest months of my life with MS:

"Fall seven times, stand up eight."

from urick to becoming jennifer digmann

BY JENNIFER

yesterday i went to a reunion luncheon with some of my sorority sisters. it's been 12 years since i graduated from college and at least that many since i had seen most of them. during my college days, i was quite different than i am now. even my name was different.

throughout college i was known as "urick," my maiden name. that was the price we jennifers paid for being born in the '70s when jennifer was so popular. we all went by our last names. there were five of us when i became a member of delta phi epsilon sorority. We were silly, occasionally drunk college girls, so going by our last names kept us straight. until i graduated in the spring of '97, i was known mostly as urick, a name i wore with pride!

only six short months after i graduated from college, multiple sclerosis entered my life. and as awful and unkind as the disease has been, i will admit that my ms diagnosis was one of the best things to ever happen to me.

no, seriously, it was!

november 14, 1997, was one of the worst days of my life. but on that day – my ms diagnosis day – i began to put my life in order. my order began with two sentences, commands really, from my neurologist. "stop drinking for a month and stop smoking ... forever," he told me. it seemed cocktails were not going to help me deal with my disease. and he thought i didn't need to smoke and potentially add cancer to my already full plate.

those were the first two steps i took in the right direction. i quit smoking and really, i've quit drinking. because when i walked, i didn't need alcohol to make walking any more of a challenge. and even now that i don't walk, i don't need alcohol to challenge my ms-compromised bladder.

multiple sclerosis also was forcing me to grow up, stand up for myself, become, as my friend diana puts it, "my own best advocate." doctors could help me deal with this disease but i learned if i was educated about new treatments or medications, i could ask the right questions and engage in useful dialogue during necessary medical appointments. plus, doctors always called me jennifer, urick was just my last name.

also, i quickly was seeing that family and friends mattered to me the most. i learned which ones of both were going to be there for the long haul. learning how to not focus only on me and my disease has taken a while but i hope i've learned it. and i hope i'm a better daughter, sister and friend because of it. again i begrudgingly have to credit my ms.

ms also has taught me or forced me to stop sweating the small stuff and to find joy in the simple, little things. like how dan and i finally figured out how to get me on and up from the couch and also to be proud of small accomplishments because really they are not small. after all, it is a big deal when i ride my arm bike for 11 minutes.

and it is a big deal that i've lost over 100 pounds since i was diagnosed. sure, i never hit the gym and it was my ms depression that made the first 60 pretty easy to lose. but without discipline, a supportive husband and weight watchers, this recent 55 lb. loss wouldn't be possible. and really none of it would have happened without ms motivating me.

but hands down, the number one reason i'm thankful for my ms is because multiple sclerosis was what brought dan and me together at the "finding your buried treasure" program. and since our wedding day september 10, 2005, i've proudly been known as jennifer digmann.

p.s. what's really cool is that one of my sisters didn't even recognize me because i look "so skinny!" and i thank ms for that.

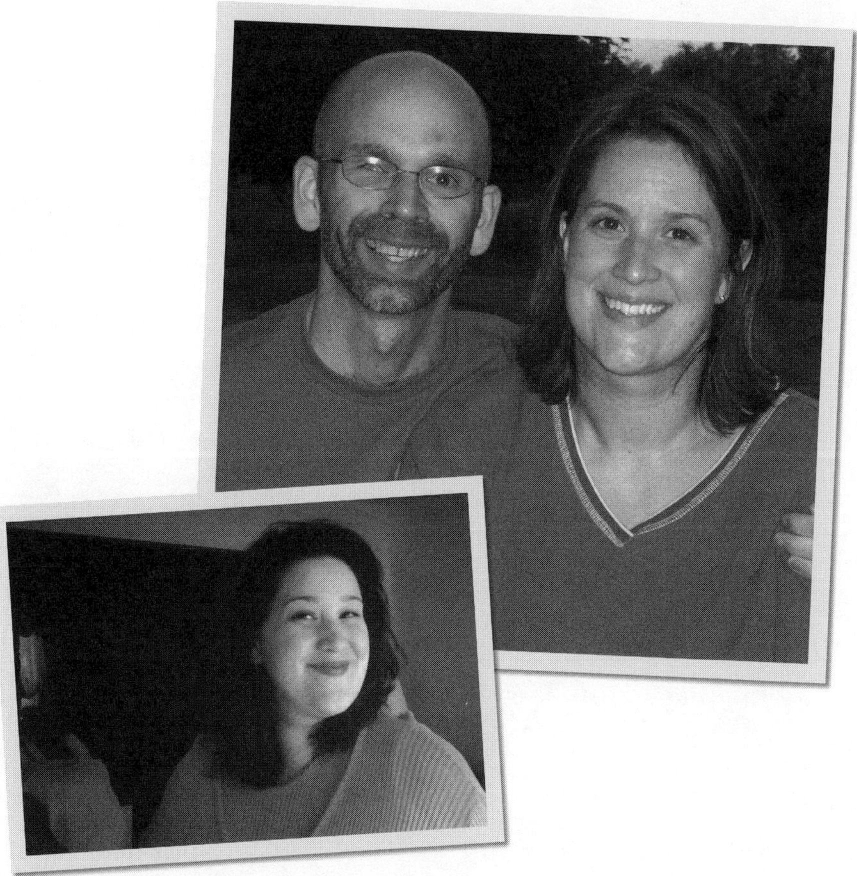

Guilty as charged

BY DAN

For the second time this year, a sense of longing weakens me as I watch the people running along the streets. I can't do that. Another calf muscle tear has set me back a step or two; no longer able to run ... right now.

Give it time. Recover. Go for a walk instead.

My runner mindset cringes at the thought of going for a walk. Yay. A walk. It'll take me twice as long to cover half the distance of my regular run. I won't even work up a sweat, so it's barely worth the effort or the time I'll put into it. Such sour grapes. That's the runner whining.

My anger soon gets a shot of reality when I think of Jennifer and others living with the same disease I have who only wish they could walk a tenth of the distance as me in 10 times the amount of time. And I wonder if they are weakened by a similar sense of longing every time they watch people walking along the streets. They can't do that. Time and wicked MS exacerbations set them back a step or two; no longer able to walk ... right now.

Take the time. Remember. Fake a smile instead.

I only hope I'll never know what that's like.

I pray I can recapture my strength and run. Push myself, train and enter a race. Throw my previous personal-best times out the window and set a new mark for me today. See my name and time in the race results; concrete proof that I still can put my best foot forward and stride across the finish line.

I only wish Jennifer could know what that's like.

For us, I walk on with a renewed sense of grateful determination. And with every step I praise and curse this disease for what it's doing: forcing us to be content with what we still have left, only to feel guilty for selfishly wanting more.

He warned me

BY JENNIFER

Seven years ago my neurologist at the time reluctantly gave me a prescription for a wheelchair. "When I give my patients this, they almost never walk again," he told my mom and me.

"But doctor," I said, "I plan on walking for a long time. Don't worry. It's just that right now, I'm so tired. And I'm especially tired of falling down. And lately I've been missing out on so much. You understand that, right?" I was naively asking a middle-aged doctor to sympathize for the lost social life of a 27-year-old woman.

"Besides, a wheelchair is just another way to get around. It's not like I'm planning to use it every day. It'll only be for navigating long distances, like parking lots at concerts or ball games, maybe lengthy shopping trips even, but it's only for convenience. You know, conserve my energy."

He listened quite patiently but he still had his doubts. I just couldn't understand why he was so opposed to me owning my own wheelchair. After all, didn't he want me to be comfortable? Or at least safe?

In these seven years since that conversation, I have come to understand his reluctance. He was opposed because he knew my short-term reasons were overlooking the long-term realities of life in a wheelchair.

When I began using my chair, I started to believe that I had outsmarted and proven him wrong. After all, I was walking 80 percent of the time and wheeling the other 20 percent. Not a bad arrangement, I thought.

But over time the balance subtly shifted. I missed the slow development of my reliance on the wheelchair because I was so impressed by how much I could accomplish when using it.

"Look at me go," I remember thinking. "This disease is no match for me."

Ahh. Silly, silly me! Sadly, I realize now that unused muscles atrophy.

Despite regular and intense physical therapy to strengthen my weakened muscles, I remained comfortable and safe from falls as I depended more and more on my chair. And my weakened, unused muscles led to pain – and nobody likes pain, especially me – so my chair kept the pain at bay. It really is a vicious cycle.

Sometimes I think the worst thing about my Multiple Sclerosis is that the disease has left me completely dependent on a wheelchair. But in reality the absolute worst part of my MS is the almost constant guilt I live with. I often feel as though I gave up. Really. Especially during my irrational, emotional moments. (Be honest: We ALL have them, MS or not.)

Unfortunately, I carry this guilt, frustration and sadness with me. Yes, I try to stuff it down. Silence it. But it's almost always there.

However, in a logical frame of mind, I know that it was this chronic disease that took away my ability to walk. It's just so easy to feel guilty, or sorry for myself, and I understand now why my neurologist was so opposed to writing that prescription.

OK. I've learned my lesson. Joke's over. I think I'll start walking again. Can I have my do-over now? Unfortunately life doesn't work like that. In her book, *On Death and Dying,* Elizabeth

Kubler Ross writes about the five stages of death, which are denial, anger, bargaining, depression and acceptance. Almost daily I deal with my MS by angrily bargaining with God. Fruitless, I know. Life just doesn't work like that.

But, I try to accept the death of my ability to walk. In doing that, I realize I'm far too accepting of the death of my walking. Life just shouldn't work like that. Isn't giving up hope of walking just plain giving up? I'm not giving up to anyone, anything. Especially MS.

Starting today I'm making a conscious choice to reclaim the possibility of walking. I know it is going to be difficult and frustrating. But while it may not happen, I'm realizing that I'll die before I accept that I will never walk again.

A race for my record book

BY DAN

I told Jennifer I'd be happy if I finished the 8K at Flint's Crim Festival of Races in under 50 minutes.

That was going to average out to a 10-minute-per-mile pace. This was slower than my normal pace, but I never had run a race of this distance. Plus, I had heard horror stories about the "Bradley hills" along this route that have challenged even the most elite of runners – of which I am not.

So, yeah, I was going to be happy if I finished the 5-mile route in 50 minutes.

Jennifer and her dad, Vic, had made it up to the finish line at about the 48-minute mark to cheer me through the chute. (I always shut off my iPod when the finish line is in sight so I can hear her encouraging voice.)

Minutes passed by and they hadn't seen me finish the race. Jennifer was getting worried because she's from Flint, and she knows what the Bradley hills are like.

At the 60-minute mark they started to talk about how they were going to have to be very supportive because I was going to be disappointed that I didn't finish as well as I had hoped.

About this time, they saw me coming ... up the sidewalk with my hands full of the bottles of water I got at the finish line some 14 minutes earlier. I had made it to the finish line before they did.

I finished the race in 43 minutes, 47 seconds – an average per-mile pace of 8 minutes, 49 seconds. Turns out this time placed me 9th out of 31 runners in my age group and 166th out of more than 750 runners in the 8K race.

And I've had MS for nearly a decade.

Jennifer, who like me still is beaming with pride with how well I did, asked me what I remember most about my first 8K. It wasn't the Bradley hills, which I told her were, "A piece of cake." Instead, I never will forget getting choked up when I turned the corner onto the bricks of the downtown Flint street and saw the blue banner stretching over the finish line: I was going to finish this race and was going to finish it in a time faster than I ever dreamed possible.

As I moved forward with everything I had left in my body, I remembered the incident earlier this year that had me running scared. How easy it would have been to give up on running (and coincidentally myself), which in turn would have given MS an undeserved victory.

With my faith, family, friends and die-hard determination, I stuck with it and kept fighting. And today, MS, victory is mine.

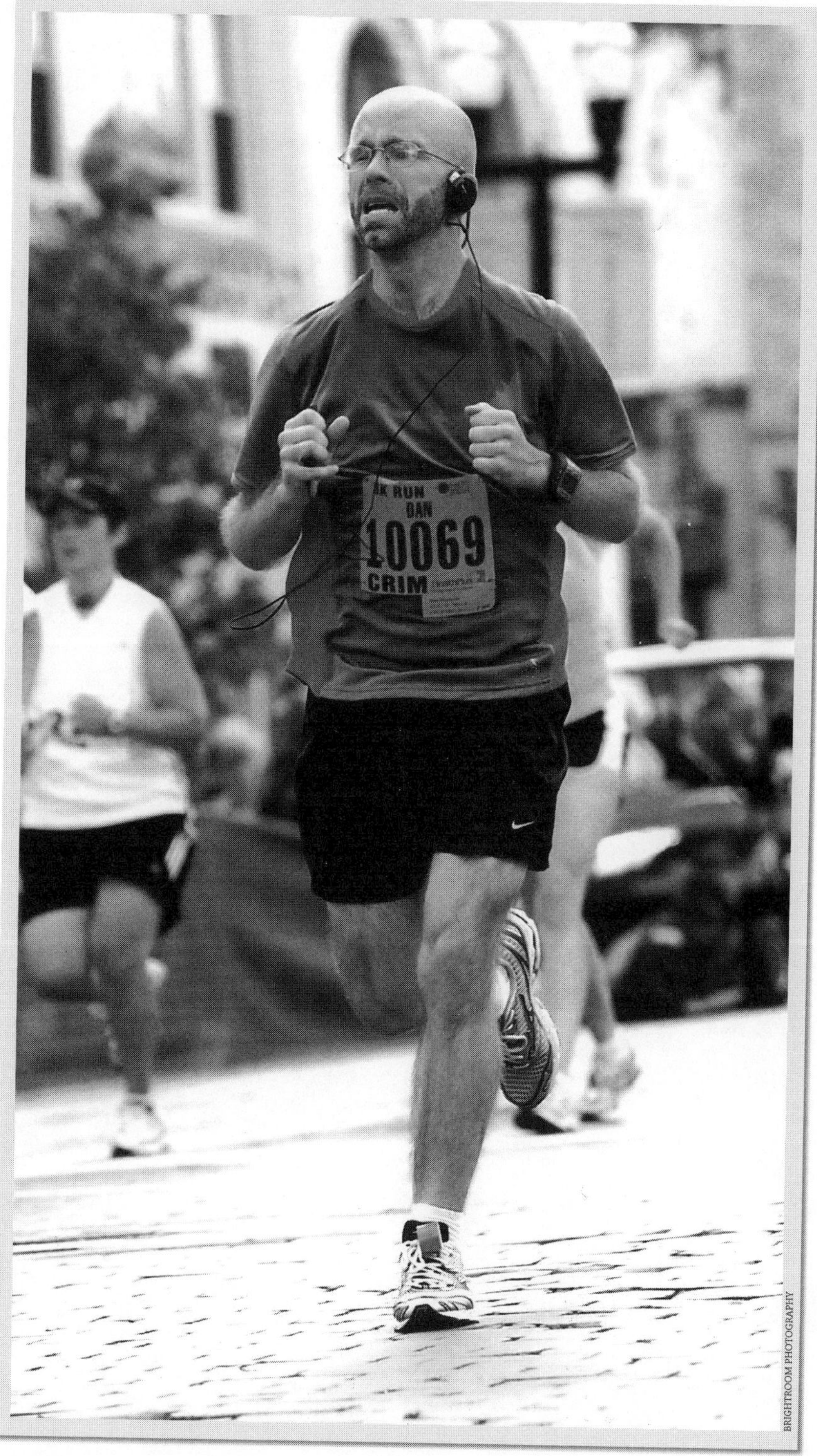

BRIGHTROOM PHOTOGRAPHY

Enough of that question

BY JENNIFER

Happy Holidays and Happy New Year!

Have you enjoyed the last week? Busy celebrating with family and friends, I bet. So are you like me – and I believe most Americans are – a person who celebrates with food?

Well my holidays were wonderful, but I'll be honest with you: I've been celebrating since Halloween. Somehow, it's all been downhill since then.

First it was, "One little piece of candy won't hurt," then, "Oh I shouldn't, but what's Thanksgiving without at least a sliver of pumpkin pie?" Then to Christmas and two words: cream puffs. My mom, Pam, makes the most delicious cream puffs from scratch! Come to discover, most of the people I've been celebrating with are great cooks.

Weight Watchers never had a chance, and thus the question I'm growing tired of: "Are you still doing Weight Watchers?"

First time I heard that, my answer was, "Yep! I'm still down 55 pounds," and I said it with pride. Sure, there was a little voice in the back of my head saying, "Not for much longer if you don't watch it," but it was pretty easy to ignore. After all, I still was going to WW meetings and being somewhat mindful of a healthy diet.

However, the last time someone posed this question, I couldn't say much. It was weeks since I had last attended a meeting, no boasting about my weight loss total. Instead I blushed, fidgeted uncomfortably and stammered, "I'm looking forward to starting again in the New Year."

Well, here it is. And here I am – a place I've been before, but I can't believe I'm here again. I must lose weight! Not just for appearance or clothes fitting properly or even for my health so much.

But it's for Dan and my caregivers and for what I still have that my MS hasn't taken from me: my ability to stand and make transfers. Managing my weight is something I still can control. I find comfort in food but what comfort is food when Dan can't lift me or my caregivers complain of having sore backs?

Gaining weight is selfish, and that's where my MS is both a blessing and a curse. It's a blessing because it gives me a very good reason to lose weight. It makes me realize that I function day-to-day with help; help that I want and need to lose weight for. It's a curse because losing weight no longer is a choice I make on my own. The disease is indirectly calling the shots.

But any way you slice it, I am going to lose weight in 2010, for Dan, my caregivers, and most importantly, for me. And as much as Dan hates it when I say it, I am so back on the horse!

Anyone want to get on their horse and ride along with me?

PSA from Jennifer

BY JENNIFER

If you ever have reason to stop walking (like you really have a choice in the matter), here are a few things to think about and realities to be prepared for. This may be construed as a "feeling sorry for myself" kind of essay, but really I just want to prepare you for the reality of life in a wheelchair, God forbid you are ever faced with it.

No, seriously. I wish someone would have told me some of these things before I had to find them out the hard way. I think it may give people motivation to AVOID the chair as long as possible, if that's even realistic. And this is the first thing you should prepare yourself for:

- You may always wonder what you did to get yourself here, or ask "why me?" Those thoughts are normal. Frustrating, but normal. Try to look forward, not backward. Good advice! Maybe I should take it, huh?
- There may never be a day when you are not angry about how bad this sucks ... but what was that advice again? Yep, I know, the windshield is bigger than the rearview mirror. Try to move on. Accept the occasional pity parties and go forward.
- Hope others cut you slack and understand that this is a BIG loss to adjust to.
- While sitting down may look enjoyable to some, when you do it 24/7, you may get a little testy to comments like, "Oh, I sure wish I had one of those today!" (i.e. a wheelchair, scooter, or

handicapped parking permit). But at least you are not being ignored.

- Bright side. Always look for a bright side. Sometimes it's still pretty darn dark but realize something is better than nothing. You can find the bright side if you look hard enough.
- First sign of a pressure sore? Treat it! Nothing to take lightly (trust me).
- Purple is a pretty color, but just not for legs that hang down all day. Always be mindful of and kind to your circulatory system.
- Accept that people may think they are helping you with preventative medicine ("Um, no really, I want to keep my toenails!!") or by offering you unneeded help (buttoning your coat, carrying things, etc.). However, they never had a handy list like this telling them how to deal with the disabled.
- Hugs will NEVER be the same, but on the bright side, at least you're getting hugged.
- It will be OK. Different perhaps, but it will be OK. Or, at times, even better than OK.
- You will never stop hoping for a cure. That's the reality, but how are you going to make it better? After all, YOU are the one in the chair. Be your own best advocate. Make it better.

Thanks for letting me get that out. I hope it helps. Really, I intended this rant to benefit you. Truly we are all in this together, even if at times you feel all alone.

5

Pay It Forward

So many stepped up
generously lent a hand
when I needed help.

Generosity
in others humbles me
sets a high standard.

I will be seeking
appropriate avenues
to pay it forward.

–JUDY WILLIAMS

Bug bites

BY DAN

A bug usually bites me a couple times each year, but its most recent nip was somewhat venomous. Try as I may, I can't seem to stop scratching the mark it left.

It's like any other bug bite: Each time the bite itches, I scratch it. Again. And again, and again, and again.

It's close to summertime, so it's natural to think something like a mosquito bit me. But it's bigger than that. This bug bite has driven me to take my concerns from the local city council to the Michigan State Capitol Building in Lansing and just today to Capitol Hill in Washington, D.C.

It's the Advocacy Bug, and it's bitten me bad.

Inspired by our friend and National MS Society Michigan Chapter research advocate Diana Hohn, Jennifer and I encourage fellow self-help group members to be their own best advocates. We say that nobody knows your personal situations and circumstances better than you, and you need to help your cause by making your voice heard and opinions understood.

I'm doing what I can to inform my elected officials of the issues I'm passionate about and encourage them to wholeheartedly consider taking action on behalf of me, Jennifer and the more than 400,000 other Americans living with Multiple Sclerosis.

I got started many years ago when Cathy Zuker, leader of the Isabella County MS self-help group, introduced me to presenting to members of the local city council a resolution proclaiming May as MS Awareness Month within their jurisdiction. So we did and at one point, our group succeeded in having five local governments within Gratiot County passing such a resolution.

While such an effort wasn't going to change the world, our elected officials saw the local faces of MS, knew such a disease was prevalent in their communities, and no longer were oblivious to our realities when they conducted business for the city and county.

Then the Advocacy Bug bit a little harder, and Jennifer and I learned the value of meeting with our state legislators in Lansing at Older Michiganians Day to advocate for funding that supports the Medicaid MI Choice Waiver Program. This invaluable program provides Jennifer the assistance she needs for daily living activities while I continue to work full time at Central Michigan University. When we recently participated in our fourth-ever such event we had the opportunity to meet our newly elected officials Rep. Kevin Cotter and Sen. Judy Emmons. What a rush!

Just yesterday I scratched an advocacy itch that took my voice all the way to the nation's capitol. Through the National MS Society's Action Alert, I learned of the need to write my senators and encourage them to support those living with MS by signing onto a bipartisan Dear Colleague letter circulated by Sen. Sheldon Whitehouse (RI) and Sen. Mike Johanns (NE) that urges the Appropriations Committee to direct a similar proportion of funds toward the MS research program in the Congressionally Directed Medical Research Programs (CDMRP) as compared to the past three federal funding cycles.

And so, with technical language that the Action Alert provided, I added some of my personal experiences and perspectives and sent the letter to Michigan Sen. Debbie Stabenow and Sen. Carl Levin. In addition, I followed up with sending emails to notify Sen. Whitehouse and Sen. Johanns that I had contacted my senators to support their efforts.

In addition to hearing back from a staff member in Sen. Johanns' office, a staff member in Sen. Whitehouse's office emailed me to share the final appropriations letter "hot off the presses!" She wrote, "As you will see, Sen. Stabenow agreed to sign on – much thanks to advocates like yourself."

Again, what a rush!

And it all started with the itch to be my own best advocate and make sure our voices are heard.

Awesome advocacy experiences

BY DAN

Jennifer and I, along with her care coordinator Rochel Genge, R.N., and others from Region VII Area Agency on Aging interacted with many elected state officials at the third annual Older Michiganians Day in Lansing.

We even have photographic proof that we advocated for the MI Choice Medicaid Waiver Program through impromptu conversations with influential legislators Sen. John Gleason, Sen. Deb Cherry and Sen. Roger Kahn on the lawn in front of Michigan's State Capitol Building. While we have met Sen. Cherry and Sen. Kahn before, this was the first time we met Sen. Gleason.

Jennifer followed up with Sen. Gleason after he spoke to the more than 600 OMD participants to thank him for supporting the Medicaid Waiver Program.

But we forever will get giddy when we think and talk about our chance meeting for which we have no picture. No picture because we never expected to run into our State Rep. Bill Caul in the House Office Building hallway as he was rushing to get to a meeting in the Capitol Building across the street.

Sure, we were on our way up to his office to remind him of the MI Choice Waiver Program and how it saves the state millions of dollars and how it is making it possible for Jennifer – one of his constituents – to continue living in her own home and positively contributing to her community. But as we made our way to get in line for the elevator, Rep. Caul made his way around the hallway corner and I whispered to Jennifer, "That's Bill Caul right there!"

Jennifer made a split-second pause to increase the speed of her power wheelchair and, without saying a word to me, sternly rolled forward and called out, "Excuse me, Rep. Caul?"

The noticeably tall representative who has served our district since 2004 stopped, looked down at Jennifer and smiled.

"I don't know if you remember me, but we've been down here before to advocate for the MI Choice Medicaid Waiver Program that provides the services for me to continue living in my own home ..." Rep. Caul was shaking his head and kindly cut Jennifer off.

"Of course I remember you," he said with a smile.

Perhaps he says this to all his constituents but we've never felt someone, especially a politician, offer such a genuine confirmation that he knew who we were. They say pictures are worth a thousand words, and I'm wondering if the reason we have no picture of our meeting with Rep. Caul is because a thousand words wouldn't be enough to describe this moment.

Knowing he had to get going, Jennifer told him we would leave some MI Choice information in his office. While he needed to get going, Rep. Caul stood there for a few more seconds to thank us for coming and for what we do to advocate for the needs of Michigan's elderly and disabled citizens.

He shook our hands and then made it to his session a few minutes late, all because he took the time to listen to what we had to say.

We came home feeling so empowered and excited about the work we had done that day.

But it not only was for the work we had done to help ourselves, it was knowing our efforts also helped the people who weren't able to be there to speak for themselves.

We always tell members of our MS self-help group they should find their passion and be voices to make things better for themselves and for others like them. For example, if advocating for the needs of people living with MS is your passion, a great place to start is registering for the National MS Society's Action Alert to receive news and information about MS advocacy news and legislative issues.

To borrow the line that our respected fellow blogger Michael Gerber uses to conclude each of his posts at *Perspective is Everything*: "Participate. Make a difference. Live a life that matters."

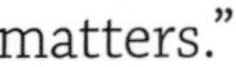

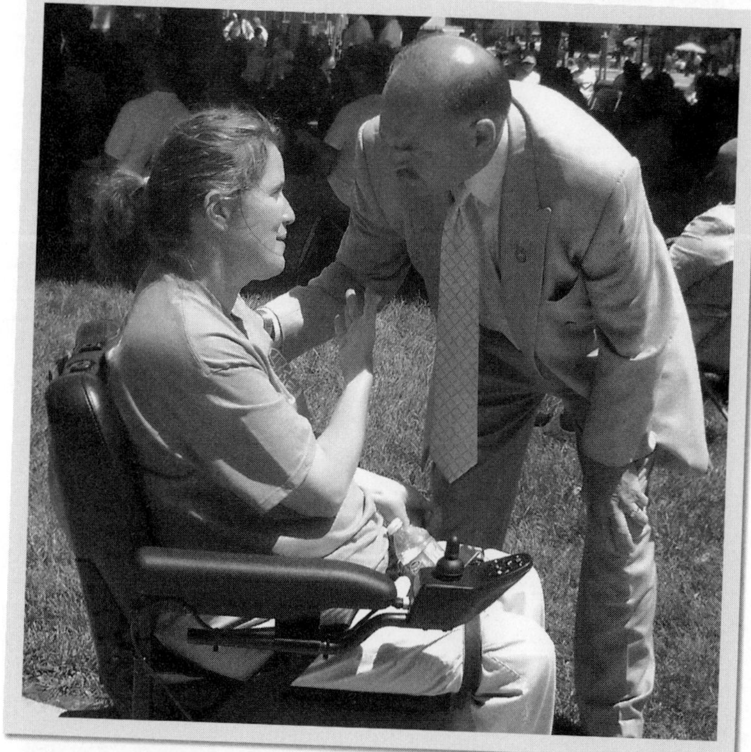

'Thank you, Sen. Kahn and members of the committee …'

BY JENNIFER

There Dan and I were, sitting at the table with two microphones, testifying before six Michigan senators.

Dan was to my left and a gallery of about a hundred people sat behind us (thank God they were sitting behind us!) and listened to what we had to say.

The Region VII Area Agency on Aging had asked if we'd be willing to testify before a Michigan Senate Appropriations Subcommittee about our experiences with the MI Choice Medicaid Waiver Program.

When they asked, we jumped (OK, not me because of that wheelchair thing) at the chance to share our story. We often say to our MS support group, "Be your own best advocate." So when we were given this chance to speak to our legislators, we had to practice what we preach.

And it was WONDERFUL!

We had the floor for about two minutes to tell how this program helps us to live our life together. How incredible that these senators, namely Sen. Roger Kahn and Sen. Deb Cherry, personally thanked us for coming, saying that it was nice to see the faces of the people MI Choice is helping.

Thanks to Region VII that coordinates the caregivers who help me, many of our state legislators had already seen our faces and knew our story. The agency recently featured us on a poster displayed at a Michigan Legislative Luncheon in Lansing. And it wasn't just a little poster. It was 2- by 3-foot displayed right there on the welcome table.

We hope that our story helps demonstrate to our state senators and representatives how this valuable program truly benefits so many people, as well as the state of Michigan. With this, we're even more excited about following up with our legislators each year at Older Michiganians Day.

My Home is MI Choice
For Jennifer & Dan Digmann
Life as a "normal" married couple because of the MI Choice Medicaid Waiver...
PRECIOUS.
Choice is the future of Long-Term Care.
Expanding community-based service options for seniors and the disabled has saved Michigan $178 million in the past 7 years.
REGION VII AREA AGENCY ON AGING

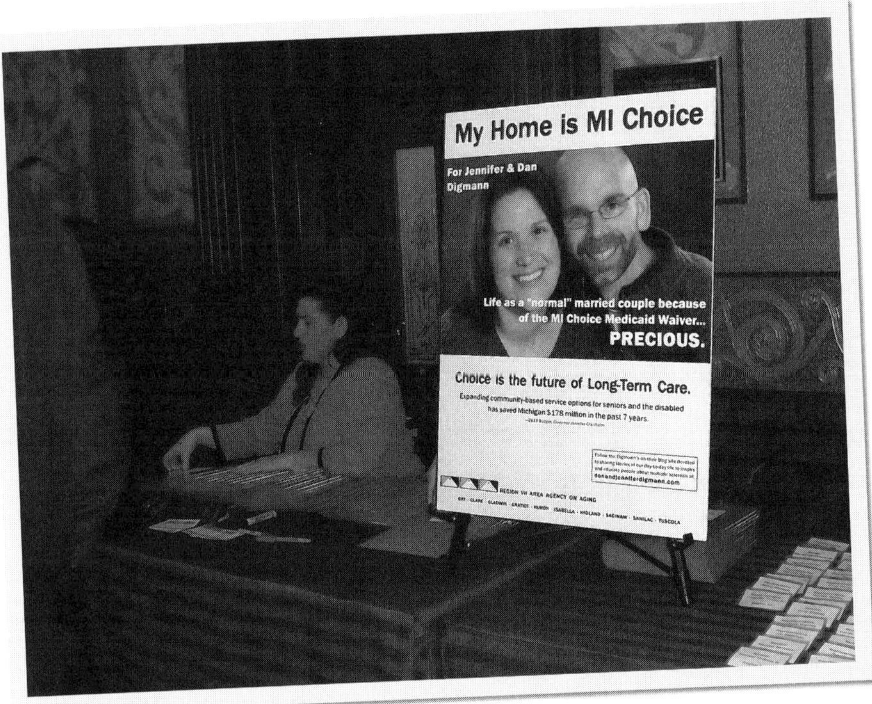

Our once-in-a-lifetime experience

BY DAN AND JENNIFER

Never again will Jennifer and I be able to tell this story about our experiences in the days leading up to and during the 2009 Walk MS.

Our backyard and house were converted into a movie set of sorts, complete with a director, cameraman, lights, cameras and a sunlight reflector thingy you see on many outdoor Hollywood sets. Not to mention that on several occasions, a neighbor passing by could have heard the words: "And ... action!" echoing across the yard.

i felt like such a star! i have what i consider a pretty ordinary life. it's a good life, but it's ordinary ... i'm just living. but for two days i had cameras pointing at me, a director asking me questions and people caring about what i had to say. and it felt amazing!

We're still humbled and overwhelmed by the fact that we were one of three nationwide winners in the Acorda Therapeutics "I Walk Because" podcast contest. Acorda is one of the Walk MS sponsors and through its "I Walk Because" campaign was looking for people with MS to tell their story – in their own words – about why they walk and what Walk MS means to them.

to find these people, acorda launched a nationwide contest inviting all walk ms registrants to submit a 30-second video about why they should be chosen to tell their story. the winners will tell their story as part of a video series that soon will be broadcast on acorda's "i walk because" website.

We felt that because we're married and both are living with MS, we'd have a great story to share. Fortunately through the video we made (thanks Cynthia and Wes!) Acorda did too.

in our winning video submission i say that i walk because i can't walk and want to make sure dan always can, and dan says that he walks because he can and that hopefully through our effort with walk ms, someday i might be able to walk again. awwww. it was very sweet!

This theme carried through into the on-camera conversations we had in our video shoot, and we are soooo excited to see what Joe (the director), Darren (the skateboarding cameraman) and the production crews with StudioPMG and Acorda Therapeutics put together! They got everything from interviewing us and getting

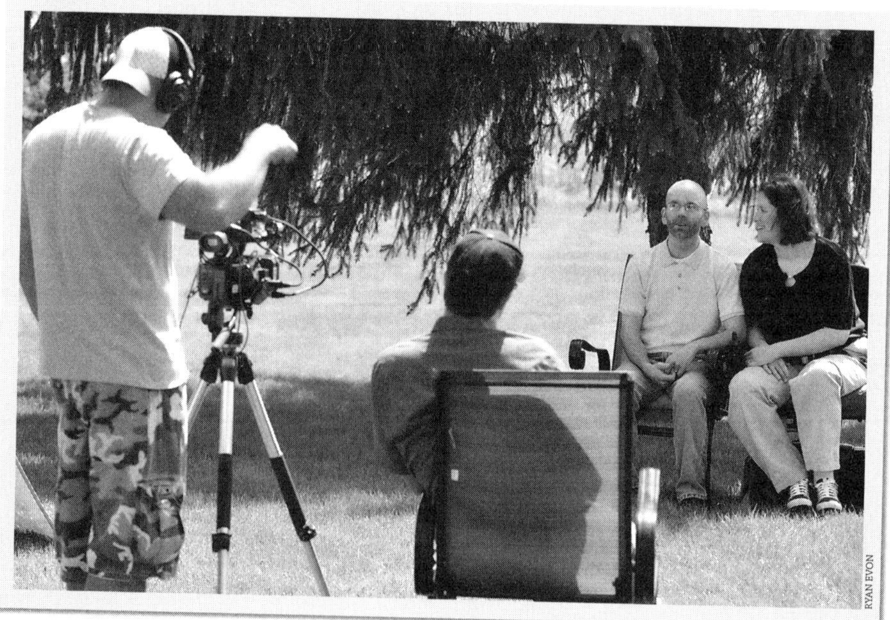
RYAN EVON

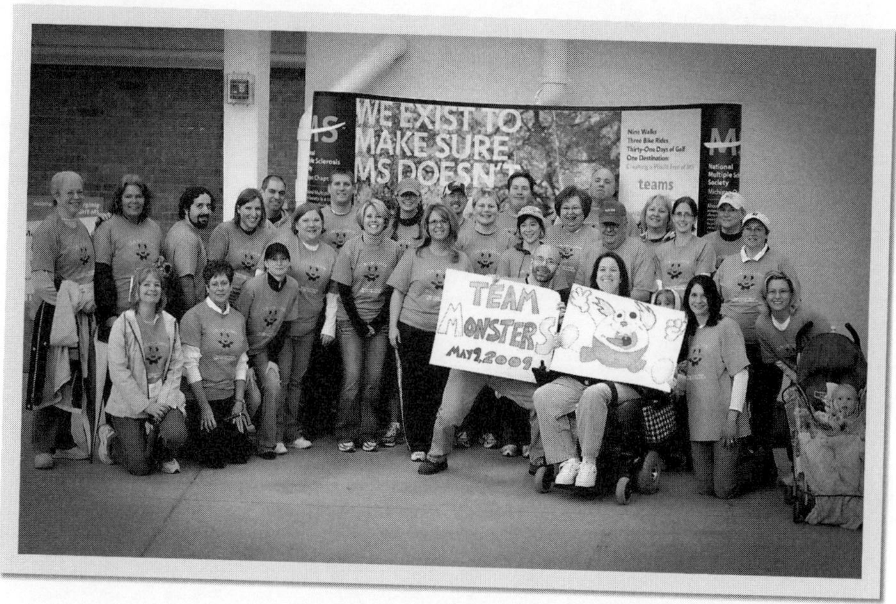

footage here at home to following us and members of our team – Team MonsterS – at the walk in Frankenmuth.

we're hoping the final podcast will be posted for the whole world to see within the next several weeks.

BTW: Our "I Walk Because" podcasts are available online at http://tinyurl.com/digmannpodcast

And it's all because we have MS

BY DAN AND JENNIFER

So Jennifer and I are sitting here still reeling from a flurry of weekend Walk MS events. Certainly, participating in the MS walk to increase awareness about Multiple Sclerosis and raise money to support MS research and programs is an event we look forward to every year.

but even though this was the seventh year we've walked together with team monsters at the walk in frankenmuth, this was unlike anything we've ever done before. first of all, it isn't every year the national ms society asks me to be a power partner to say a few words at the starting line, umm no pressure.

Jennifer did an incredible job as a Power Partner getting the walkers fired up and convincing them that the early morning rain was going to stop.

and i promised the walkers that there would be no need for umbrellas.

And if Jennifer was feeling any pressure addressing the thousands of people at the walk, she didn't show it. I imagine she, like me, had gotten used to being watched. After all, we had just spent the day before the walk with a two-man production crew from StudioPMG in Irvine, Calif., who was interviewing us and getting footage for our Acorda Therapeutics national contest-winning podcast.

darren and joe are two of the nicest guys we'll ever meet, and we are so looking forward to seeing what they develop for the podcast that soon will appear on acorda's "i walk because" website.

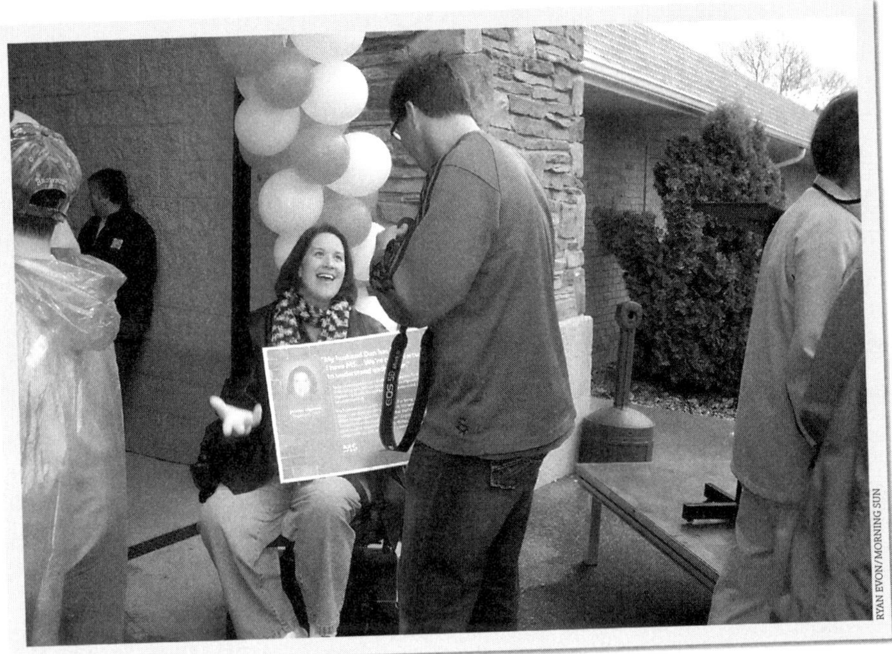

RYAN EVON/MORNING SUN

they continued following us at the walk – joe on foot with his digital camera and darren on skateboard with his video camera – filming us and asking more questions. not to be forgotten was ryan, a modern day kato from *the pink panther*, hiding amongst trees and on bridges taking our picture for a photo story he's developing for the local newspaper, morning sun.

While the media attention was an exciting one-of-a-kind element of our walk experience this year, the continued support of our family and friends is what made the weekend's event as meaningful as ever for us. There's something indescribably humbling about the amount of support we receive from our loved ones for the walk, as well as throughout each day of the year.

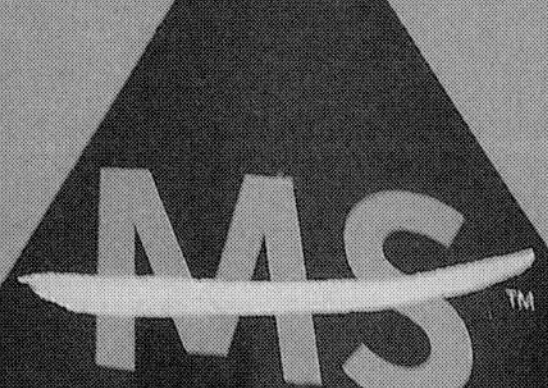

RYAN EVON/ MORNING SUN

Were they really talking about us?

BY DAN

After presenting eight of the 10 awards, Matt "Mojo" Lersch paused to ask officials for direction before moving onto the ninth.

The master of ceremonies at the National Multiple Sclerosis Society, Michigan Chapter's 2009 Annual Meeting and Celebration of Volunteers and Top Fundraisers in Livonia showed the crowd of nearly 200 people the specific directions typed in the script he was following.

"This award is a secret," whispered Mojo, who hosts the Rock 'N Roll Sideshow on Lansing's Rock Station Q106 and was diagnosed with MS in December 2008. "Only a few people know who's getting it."

Mojo then was given the green light to present the 2009 MS Achievement Award, which expresses the NMSS' appreciation of and to provide recognition to an individual with MS who has achieved outstanding success in life.

He described that while the award recipient doesn't need to be an NMSS member or volunteer, this person must have made a significant impact in his or her profession and community.

But when Mojo began to read about the accomplishments of this year's "secret" recipient, he led with, "This couple ..." And we soon realized he was talking about us.

Our eyes pooled with tears and the reality quickly sank in: We were being named the 2009 MS Achievement Award recipients.

In following what has become a built-in emotional defense mechanism for us, we held each other's hand and both started

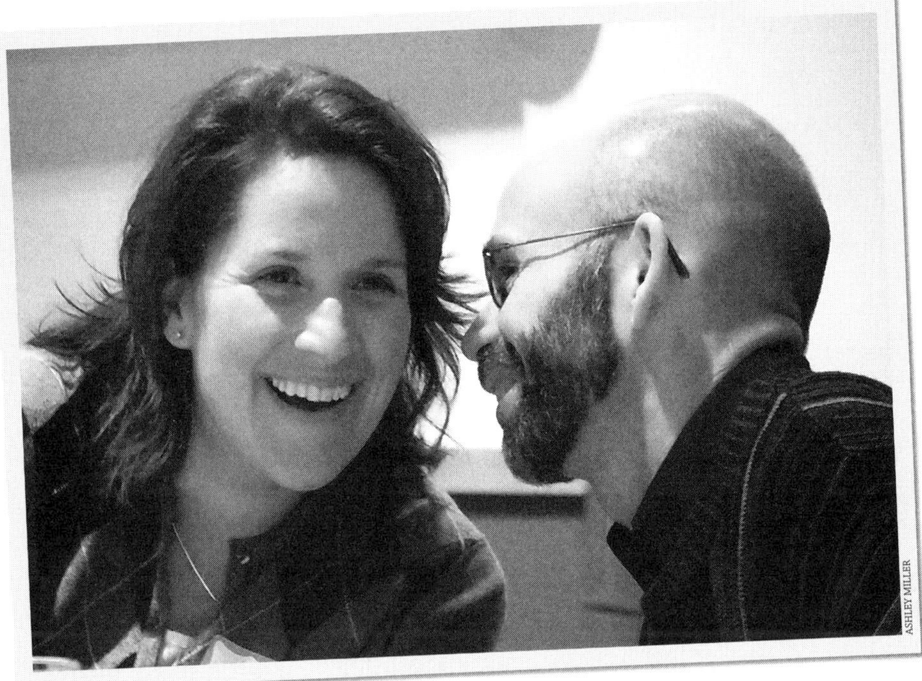

ASHLEY MILLER

laughing to keep from crying. We were so surprised to be recognized for what we've done to increase awareness about MS, we didn't even make it on stage to receive the award.

Were they really talking about us? It took NMSS Michigan Chapter President Elana Sullivan meeting us at the foot of the stage with the award for us to believe that this really happened.

It's incredibly overwhelming and humbling to be recognized like this. After all, we never asked for this disease. We are just doing what we can to get the word out about MS and help people positively move forward when dealing with whatever challenges they face.

Through our volunteering at NMSS events, public speaking and maintaining our blog, we hope to increase awareness and public understanding of this chronic disease of the central nervous system that affects us and more than 400,000 people nationwide, including 18,000 in Michigan.

This prestigious award is our proof that you never know what kind of impact your actions will make on others.

6

My Intention

Full recovery.
That will be my intention
until my last breath.

I don't want to hear
the odds are impossible.
I aim to beat them.

One thing I do know.
Giving up beforehand means
guaranteed defeat.

–JUDY WILLIAMS

What helps us through MS

BY DAN

I think my mom and dad – Nancy and Roger – will be surprised to hear that a gift they gave me more than two decades ago is something Jennifer and I turn to often in dealing with the daily realities of Multiple Sclerosis.

I'm surprised myself.

After all, when you get confirmed in the Lutheran church, it's expected that you'll receive some sort of religious memorabilia commemorating the event. You know: it usually is something like a cross to hang on your wall, a religious plaque to set on your desktop or a special coin to carry in your pocket to remind you that God loves you.

Mine was a red prayer book that has moved with me throughout Iowa and Michigan in a silver, black and white shoebox – like an honorary piece of luggage that accompanied me every time I changed my mailing address.

I always remembered *The Lutheran Book of Prayer* was in the shoebox, but it wasn't until I was diagnosed with this chronic illness that I dug out the book and took its contents to heart. Looking in the table of contents, under the heading "During Illness," I discovered the prayer that has given me the strength I need to positively move forward through my life with MS.

And now, it's a prayer that Jennifer and I adapted and read most nights before we go to bed, and we wanted to share it with you in hopes that it may provide you comfort in your life:

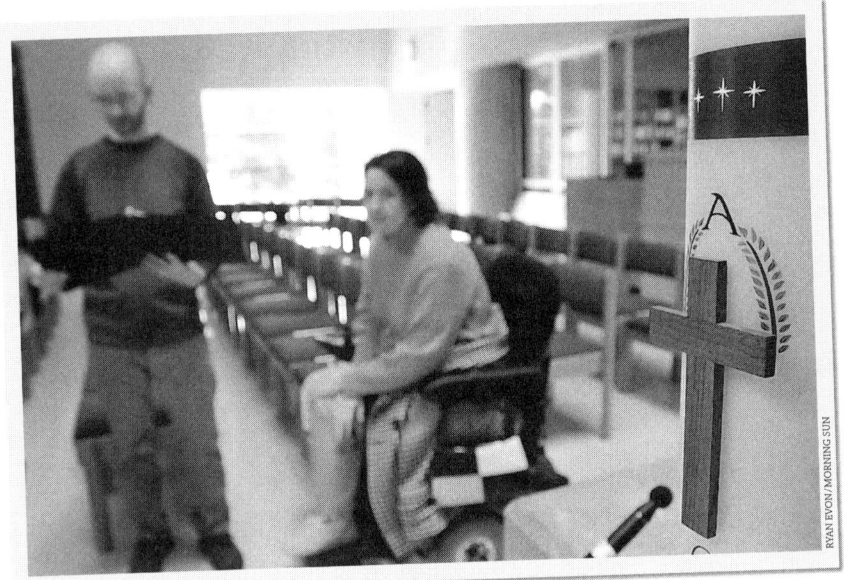

RYAN EVON/MORNING SUN

Gracious God, help Jennifer and me to accept your will in our illness. As your children we believe that you cause all things to work together for our good, both of body and of spirit. But sometimes in the midst of illness and pain we forget or doubt. Forgive our weak faith. When we become impatient, encourage us by your word. Despite our worries and suffering, help us by our lives to reflect the radiance and confidence of those certain of your promises of help. Restore us to sound health if it be your will, and enable us with new vigor and enthusiasm to serve you zealously for many years to come. Give us your Holy Spirit that we may always witness joyfully to our Christian faith before men and women, confessing that all life, on earth and in heaven, is a gift from you. O Lord, have mercy. Hear our prayer for Jesus' sake. Amen.

Since I was diagnosed with MS, I've never asked God, "Why me?" Rather, I continue to tell God, "Help me." And I've learned he's always here, I just need to be open to where he's offering a helping hand. Even if it's in a silver, black and white shoe box.

35

BY JENNIFER

Well, I guess it's time to face it. This Friday, Nov. 6, is my 35th birthday. And yes, I am freaking out about it.

I'm not exactly sure why, after all it's just a number. But 35 is just a bigger number than I care (or am prepared) to be.

Maybe it's because this birthday marks the beginning of middle age. No seriously, hear me on this: If I live to be the glorious age of 70, 35 is half of that. That's middle age ... Eeek!

Me – a middle-aged woman. When did that happen?

Plus this birthday is hard for me to deal with because lately my MS is causing me a little more headache than I'm used to. I guess I should call it a footache to be more accurate. I have my first pressure sore which is on my foot, and trust me they are just as painful as they are made out to be.

All I can think is you must be kidding me! This disease is not just happy with the fact it took my walking and my driving, now it's trying to make me miserable with pain all day.

Not only is it that, but it's making me feel sorry for myself. This is a challenge and temptation that those of us living with a chronic illness or disability face almost every day. That whole "Why me?" type of thinking, and I have to stop indulging in that kind of pointless waste of energy.

So I've compiled a list. Hopefully this list will keep me going in the dark days of middle age. Hee, hee ... that serious, dramatic, doom-filled tone helped me see how silly I'm being and made me smile :-)

Without further ado, here are 35 things that I'm thankful for:

35. Dan, of course.
34. Getting to dip my toes in the beautiful Pacific Ocean.
33. Owning a convertible back when I used to drive.
32. I have an amazing family, especially my parents (Thanks, Mom and Dad). Bonus: I love my in-laws.
31. Supportive, wonderful, hilarious friends.
30. All of my great memories from college.
29. Delta Phi Epsilon sorority and all of the great friends I made because of it.
28. Memories of my dog, Buster, and the day-to-day life with our cat, Cooper. Pets rule!!
27. The Medicaid Waiver program which makes our life better every single day.
26. *Simpsons* clouds.
25. Dan's smile and laugh.
24. Laughter altogether.
23. Dragon NaturallySpeaking.
22. The roof over my head and the clothes on my back.
21. A shiny new manicure.
20. Delicious birthday cake, and not having to count Weight Watchers points for it. Hey, it's my list and I can dream if I want to.
19. Afternoon hour-long insane phone conversations with my BB.
18. My church family at Immanuel Lutheran.
17. Summer of 1993: innocent stuff like watermelon seed fights and getting caught cheating at euchre and some other less innocent memories.

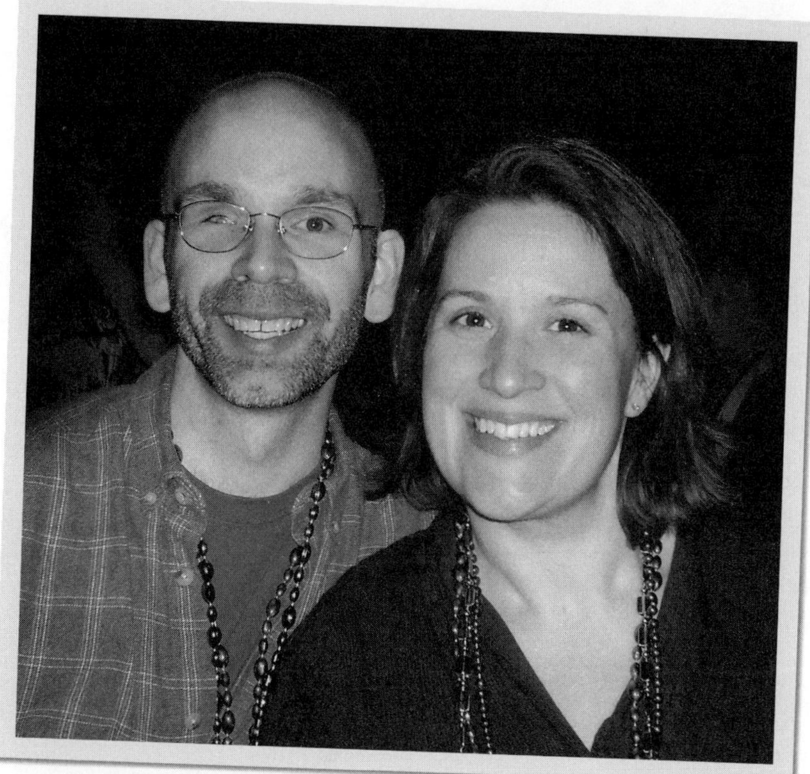

16. Good times up north with Amy at Aunt Cindy's.
15. Being able to walk when I went to Europe.
14. Heck, that I even got to take a trip to Europe!
13. Good music to chair-boogie to.
12. Clean sheets and good hair days.
11. Realizing in five years it probably won't matter (Thanks, Nora).
10. Did I mention my amazing husband, Dan, and my wonderful family?
9. The Michigan Story Festival at CMU and being able to share our story.
8. That he's not married to her anymore.
7. Fresh tomatoes in the summer.

6. No cavities at the dentist.
5. Playing a good game of Scrabble.
4. Universal design and handicapped accessible restrooms.
3. Other than having MS, Dan is in good health.
2. Other than having MS, I am in pretty good health.
1. Believe it or not, Multiple Sclerosis (after all, it helped me meet Dan and taught me to appreciate life).

This really is a pretty good list! I encourage everyone who is struggling with a dark day to make a similar list of their own. You might be surprised by everything in your life you have to be thankful for.

March Madness and life lessons

BY DAN

March Madness is in full swing, and so, talk of the Sweet 16, Final Four and Cinderella teams emerging through upsets such as No. 11 Dayton beating No. 6 West Virginia 68-60 reminds me of the Multiple Sclerosis lessons I learned on the Pine Avenue Elementary School basketball court.

For the first few months following my MS diagnosis more than nine years ago, I lived in fear and was very cautious about what and how much I did. After all, I was living with a chronic illness.

I had reluctantly strolled three blocks to the elementary school to shoot baskets. Every 10 steps or so I'd dribble the ball a couple times, which was enough for me to realize the MS-induced numbness in my hands had stripped any sort of "soft touch" I had with the basketball.

Next to the school, on the flat slab of concrete that seemed more like a really big patio than a basketball court, I experienced firsthand that my ball-handling skills weren't that great and my jump shot was a little off the mark. I was undaunted by my lost dribbles and air balls because I knew my true personal test would come from the free-throw line.

Shooting free throws is the telltale sign because it's easy to track my accuracy – or lack thereof. I always shoot 10 shots for easy percentage conversion purposes.

So I stepped up to the line. Now, I have made it a rule that I never start counting until I make one shot. SWISH! one for one

... BOINK! ... one for two.... BOINK! ... one for three ... SWISH! ... two for four ... .

That first day, I went four for 10 from the line. Forty percent. Hmmmmm. Thinking back to how I shot before my hands were all but asleep, I usually shot about 70 percent. My gosh. I had lost 30 percent accuracy. MS was getting the best of me, and I was fading fast. Next year, I thought, I'll be lucky to make two baskets.

But I wasn't meant to be a free-throw god that day. Instead, it was on that day that I began to rebound from the "glass is half empty" mentality that I had embraced the day I was diagnosed. I looked deeper and realized that I couldn't blame the disease for my 30 percent decline. The real reason I missed six of 10 free throws: I hadn't shot baskets since nearly six months earlier. Of course I was going to be rusty. That's how I am the first time out every spring. Plus, I remembered that I was never Michael Jordan to begin with.

I never attended Pine Avenue Elementary, but I learned on the school's patio-like basketball court that I shouldn't be so quick to blame MS for everything that isn't going as well as it used to. I'm not so naïve as to think that MS won't adversely affect my life, but the even greater lesson I learned on the court that day was that I shouldn't be so quick to give up on myself.

Two days later, I drained eight of 10 from the line.

Every day, I embrace

BY DAN

My days are numbered. Medical experts essentially tell me this all the time.

I heard it most recently when I attended an MS conference last weekend hosted by the University of Michigan Hospital in Ann Arbor.

In not so many words, they said that ***most*** people with Multiple Sclerosis live with the relapsing-remitting form of the disease for so long and eventually transition to the secondary-progressive form after they've had the disease for 10 years.

I hate it when I go to these kinds of things because they often provide a subtle yet very in-my-face reminder that I truly have a chronic, progressive disease. I don't blame them for their pessimistic forecasts because I realize the medical facts don't lie.

With a decade under my belt, I guess I'm living on borrowed time.

While I don't consciously think about it, I wonder if I unconsciously realize this with every step I take. Every stair I climb. Every race I run. Every shoe I tie. Every workday I complete. Every book I read. Every sentence I write.

Everything I do.

Such a reality check has the potential to throw me off my game and into a woe-is-me abyss that could consume my life. But I won't let this happen. I'm guided by the legendary charge of Coach Jimmy Valvano who said, "Don't give up. Don't ever give up."

With a decade under my belt I know I'm living on, regardless of what form of Multiple Sclerosis I have.

I consciously realize this with every challenge I face. Every obstacle I overcome. Every frustration I feel. Every battle I lose. Every battle I win. Every moment I live life to its fullest.

Every day, I embrace.

On the river without a paddle

BY JENNIFER

Like it or not, it's fall. The leaves are changing – lots have already fallen off the trees. Temperatures are dropping. The heat is on at our house. And I'm sporting sweaters way more than T-shirts. Yep, as much as I dislike it, fall is here. Which means winter is around the corner.

Depressing, isn't it?

Rather than sulk (because sulking is fruitless), I'm remembering one of my favorite memories of this summer.

It all came about because of my rambling at a church gathering that was held at a beautiful home in Mount Pleasant situated on the Chippewa River.

"You know this is the year I'm floating the river. Not sure how, but darn it, I've lived here four years and that is something I've always wanted to do!"

I just assumed that because I can no longer walk, this dream was just that. A dream.

But as I soon learned, my rambling was heard by the right people – a Can-Do Bunch of people.

One quiet Sunday this summer, our phone rang. I answered and heard, "It's a beautiful day to go canoeing and floating. What do you think? Can you meet us at 3 p.m. at Buckley's? We sure think this might be the last nice day. And Gary, Peggy, Charlie and I think we've found the perfect spot to put you in. So what do you think?!?"

After a moment, I recognized the excited voice. It was Sue – a very excited Sue. And after another moment, I realized Sue was serious. That little statement of mine a few weeks earlier was heard by her, Gary, Peggy and Charlie, and they were going to get me on that river. And I was getting on it TODAY!!!

"Really, Sue," I gulp, "Today? You want to float the river today? Like today, in five hours?"

My mind's racing: Come on tough girl, you're not scared are you? Duh! Of course, I'm scared. Think Jennifer, think. Dan, surely he'll object. He'll think it's a crazy idea too.

"Let me check with Dan, Sue. Just a sec, OK?"

"Hey Dan, Sue et al. (truly that's what I said, apparently fear brings out my slightly academic side) want to float the river today … ."

"Sure, sounds great! What time?" he calmly asks.

Um, OK. Didn't see that coming, but if Dan thinks I can do it, I probably can.

"Well it's a plan, mind if I ask Sue K. and her husband, Dave, to join us? And what does one wear when floating the river?" I quickly ask.

"Sure, call them, the more the merrier. Um, shorts are good. See you later this afternoon!" Click.

Ah, jeez, "Dan let's go get me some shorts at Target. And then, I've got to shave my legs. Yikes, we've got to hurry. I'm floating the river at 3 o'clock."

I say it again quietly to myself: I'm floating the river at 3 o'clock.

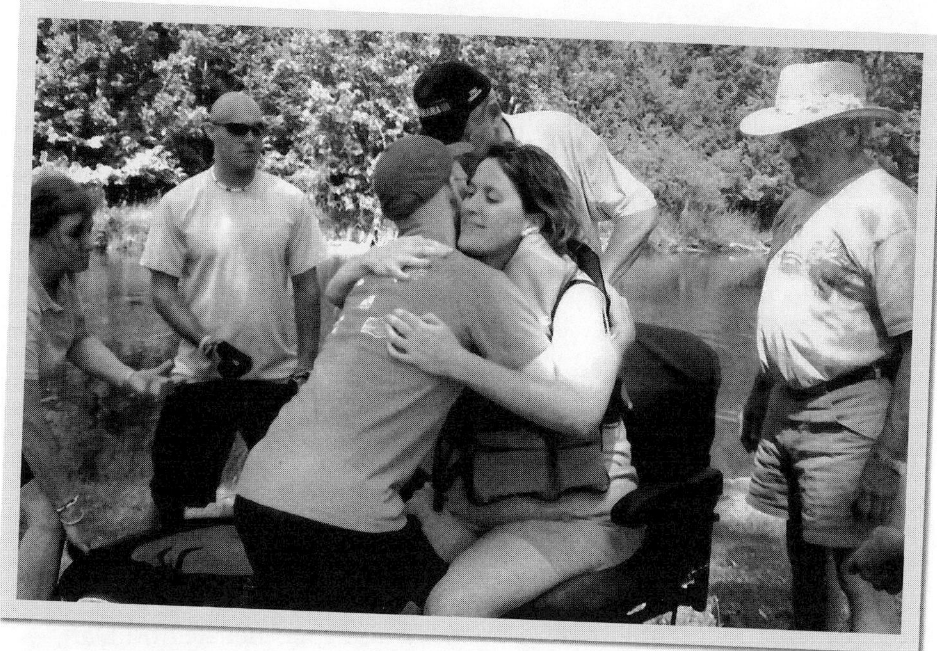

River royalty

It was a long ride to Buckley's Mountainside Canoe. While I was excited about floating the river, all that kept coming to mind were the "what if" questions: "What if I can't get in the river?" "What if I have to go to the bathroom?" "What if I get stuck on a rock?" "What if I flip over?" "What if Dan and I get separated?" And, God forbid, "What if I drown?"

Just as that last one really sunk in, Peggy jumped into our van.

"Hi, are you ready?" she asked.

Well, no I thought. I can't fully use my legs and left arm (damn MS) and you only need 4 inches of water to drown. So no, I thought, I'm not ready. Isn't it funny? Sometimes you think MS has made your life so crummy, but you soon find yourself realizing you sure would hate to lose your so-called crummy life?

"Ready as I'll ever be!" I told her confidently. I knew that these wonderful friends of mine put a great deal of effort into planning the perfect trip down the river, which was exactly what I wanted. So I put my faith in them (and God). I let it go. I trusted them all.

We left Buckley's after getting our group together and drove to the perfect spot where I could transfer from my wheelchair onto the tube and then into the river. This spot was a private residence Sue had staked out.

We all were impressed, "Gee Sue, how'd you get this perfect spot? I mean, what did you have to do to get permission to get on the river here?"

"Oh, I just asked." she said with a smile.

Dan stood me up from my wheelchair. A nice employee from Buckley's put the tube behind my back and together he and Dan, with some help from our group, gently plopped me in the tube.

I was giddy! I couldn't stop giggling and kicking my feet. "Oh my goodness, I'm really going to do this!"

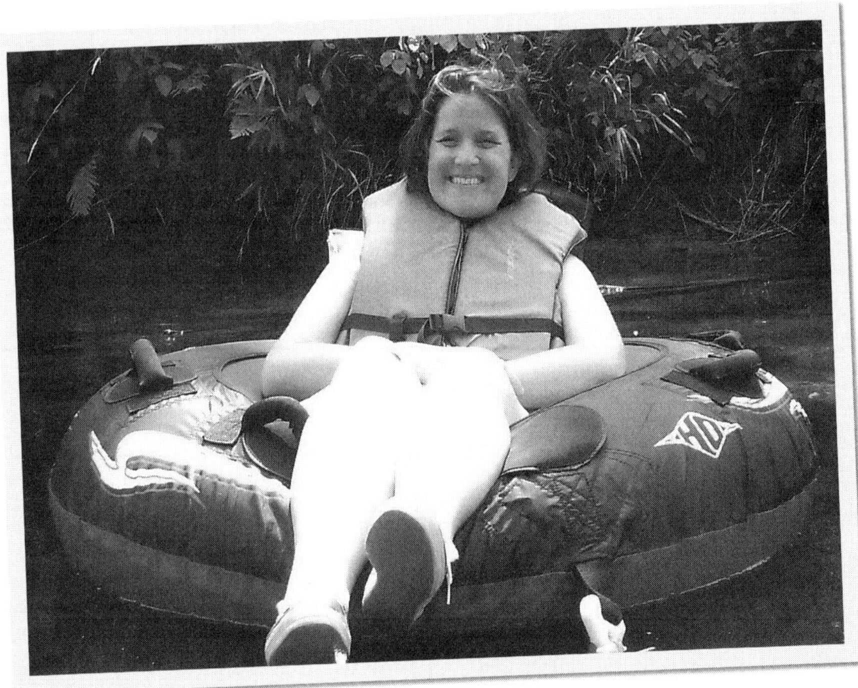

One strong, deliberate push down a little embankment and ***SPLASH***, I'm in the river. The water felt a little cold, brisk and so refreshing. Sue used a rope to tie my tube to her kayak; she was towing me down the river. The rest of our bunch got into their kayaks. I was the only one being towed and getting to float. Pretty nice, huh? And now, do you understand why I felt like royalty?

And I floated.

It was beautiful! Calm, cool water. Warm sun shining down on me. And strong, healthy, vibrant green trees lining the shore. It was so peaceful, gloriously quiet and peaceful. A feeling of just me and nature. Of course, I was with my friends and Dan, but in those few quiet moments when I wasn't shrieking, "I'm doing it! I'm really on the river," it was me and Mother Nature. It was so comforting.

For those 45 minutes that I floated the Chippewa River, I was normal. My having Multiple Sclerosis played almost no part in my floating fun. For that glorious sunny Sunday afternoon, I was on a level playing field, so to speak. My disability wasn't apparent. There wasn't a wheelchair in the water letting people in on the fact that I no longer walk. I appeared to be just as able-bodied as anyone else; I had sort of forgotten what it's like to kind of blend in. Well as blendable as a woman shouting, "I'm floating, oh wow, I'm floating!!" can be.

That afternoon was the highlight of my summer and no matter how many "thank yous" I say, they'll never be enough to thank Buckley's and my church family – The Can-Do Bunch (Sue, Gary, Peggy, Charlie, Sue K., Dave and Dan) – enough!

Magic #7

BY DAN

It's barely six songs into the set list and I'm already winded. But this is exactly what I expected from my eighth time seeing Bruce Springsteen and the E Street Band live in concert, this time promoting their *Magic* album.

I always tell my friends and family that if I could afford it, I'd buy tickets for all of them just so they could experience the nearly three hours of rock 'n roll insanity that ensues each time Springteen and his New Jersey-based posse take the stage.

Ten musicians together. At the same time. Controlled rock 'n roll chaos that only Bruce Springsteen and, in his words, "the heart-stopping pants-dropping house-rocking earth-shaking booty-quaking Viagra-taking love-making legendary E Street Band" can deliver night after night after night. For nearly three hours.

"Reason to Believe" is only the sixth song into the concert at the Palace of Auburn Hills, and I no longer can feel my hands that I've unconsciously on purpose numbed through uninterrupted applause and fist pumping. My throat is scratchy and voice is raspy from screaming the lyrics to each song as loud as I can because apparently I want Bruce and the other 18,000 people here to realize that I know every word to every song.

But not even a Springsteen freak, er, fan like me who was checking the concert logs posted on his fan-based Web site – backstreets.com – could have predicted the seventh song in his set list this night: an obscure song and concert rarity that quickly moves me to tears and makes me wish I had saved some of my voice so I could scream even louder.

"Reason to Believe" ends and then, in standard Springsteen fashion, he grunts out the cadence, "One! Two! ... One! Two! Three! Four!" and the band rips into an all-too-familiar intro. My heart stops because I realize what Bruce has pulled out of his vault.

Simply put, he plays "Jackson Cage," the third song on the first disc of *The River* album.

In January 2000, "Jackson Cage" inexplicably became the anthem, if you will, that has carried me through my life since I was diagnosed with Multiple Sclerosis. To me, nothing else describes life with MS better than this song. All you have to do is approach the song as though "Jackson Cage" is a euphemism for MS.

To this day I don't know what led me to purposely listen to this song. It was a Saturday evening, not too long after I was diagnosed. For some reason I was in the mood for the sternly commanded closing lines of the song:

Well darling can you understand
The way that they can turn a man into a stranger
To waste away down in the Jackson Cage

With lyrics in hand I listened to the song. Really listened. I began sobbing right there. Like I said earlier, all you have to do is approach the song as though "Jackson Cage" is a euphemism for MS.

You can try with all your might
But you're reminded every night
That you've been judged and handed life down in the Jackson Cage

This is so true no matter how optimistic I think I am. When I go to bed and pray at night, my hands burn from the day's activities, and I truly am reminded every night that I have MS. It's like that through the entire song.

This is the most perfect song for me when I'm having a rough MS day. It addresses the aggression and anger that comes with living with the disease, while at the same time instilling a call to stand up and fight.

It don't matter just what you say
Are you tough enough to play the games they play
Or will you just do your time and fade away down in the Jackson Cage

It's interesting to note that at this concert, when Bruce played my anthem, it actually was my wife, Jennifer, who recognized it was "Jackson Cage" before I did.

But I was the one who had tears rolling down my cheeks, screaming every lyric right with Bruce while silently thanking him for his songs that to this day still help me through, and forever will help me through, some of the toughest days of my life with this disease.

It was only the seventh song of a 23-song set list that lasted nearly three hours. But the concert could have ended there, and I would have felt I more than got my money's worth.

Halfway through

BY JENNIFER

With the posting of my Anthropology 590 grade today (a B+ and I'm OK with that), I have reached the halfway point in my Humanities graduate program at Central Michigan University.

Being in the middle, I am reflecting back on some of the things I have learned thus far in my various English, History, Film, and Anthropology classes. And because I love lists, here is my compiled "Top Ten Lessons from Graduate School."

10. Bathrooms, no matter where they are, are a major theme, setting or archetype in my life. Guess that makes the toilet a motif. At least I think that's correct. Agree? And, NEVER should any part of me be on its floor, especially my face.
9. A written in-class essay exam may sound easy enough, but living with MS for the past 13 years proved otherwise.
8. Some things may change, but procrastination rules eternal.
7. This education is excellent and the people – my professors, classmates and campus employees – are excellent plus one!
6. I do not deal with stress well. That is worth repeating: I DO NOT DEAL WITH STRESS WELL.
5. John Hughes was brilliant and *The Breakfast Club* will always be his finest work, in my humble opinion.
4. I am so lucky to be a woman living in the United States in 2010, not a woman in the American past, or a woman working in the maquiladoras of Mexico or global sex trade of Asia, Europe, the U.S. or some former Soviet republic.

3. Graduate school is tough, but nothing worth having is easy to get.
2. Freshman 15? What explains my weight gain? Hmm, #6 perhaps.
1. A CMU ALUMNI sweatshirt is such an incredible motivation tool.

And to quote Michael and Tony from *Pardon the Interruption*, "That's it. That's the list."

Pretty interesting graduate program, don't you think?

Here's looking forward to my health allowing me to complete the other half of my program, because a master's degree will be such an achievement and that shirt will be SO cute!!

The bathroom floor imprinted on my face

BY JENNIFER

Yes, on my face.

Couldn't have happened at a worse time. Or so I thought. Right there on a break from my class, Dan was helping me to pivot in the Anspach Hall bathroom and SMACK!

Profanity! Profanity! Profanity! And tears ... tears ... tears.

And that wasn't just me. I heard profanity and tears coming from Dan, too.

It was frightening, fast and so sudden. I couldn't even lift my head off the tile. I didn't even want to move and I was face down on a public bathroom floor. That's how bad it hurt.

This was supposed to be a standard trip to the bathroom. Same as we had done for each Tuesday evening over the past nine weeks of the semester. I have a regularly scheduled break during my Anthropology 590 graduate class, "Gender, Culture & Society." During this time Dan comes to the CMU campus building to help me go to the bathroom.

And it normally runs like clockwork. We get a break. We go to the bathroom. I ask if any of the women there minds if my husband comes in to help me – which they never do because women rule! – and he helps me with pivoting and transferring on and off the toilet and back into my chair.

But this night, the night before our largest speaking presentation ever, a rare miscommunication in the transfer back into my chair had me simultaneously thinking, "Timber!" and

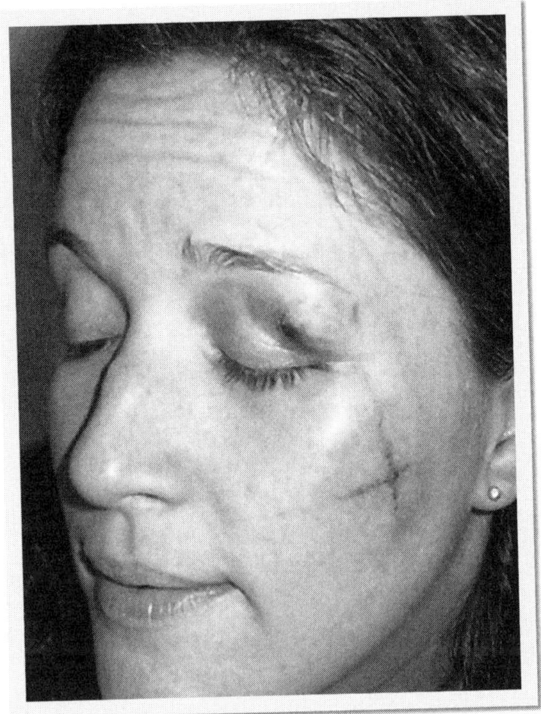

"This is going to hurt," as I fell shoulder first into the bathroom stall and then flat on my face. Thus the imprint. For real. You can see the tile lines on my cheek!

I'm lucky that there was no blood, I didn't break any teeth, and we were able to get help. (Thanks Sarah, Dr. Brown and Josh!)

I was fine once I calmed down. Dan was too. I took a couple ibuprofen and sat on the couch after my professor let me go home from class early. (Thanks again, Dr. Brown!)

And I geared up for the next day's presentations with the Women's Initiative at noon in Mount Pleasant and the Shiawassee County MS Self-help Group later that evening in Owosso.

Marked with the sign of the bathroom tile floor, Dan and I delivered two of our best speaking engagements the next day. We were fortunate enough to share our story and increase MS awareness, all while I was rockin' my first-ever black eye.

And to be frankly honest, I sported that black eye with pride because it symbolized both the reality of my Multiple Sclerosis and my determination to not let this disease hold me down.

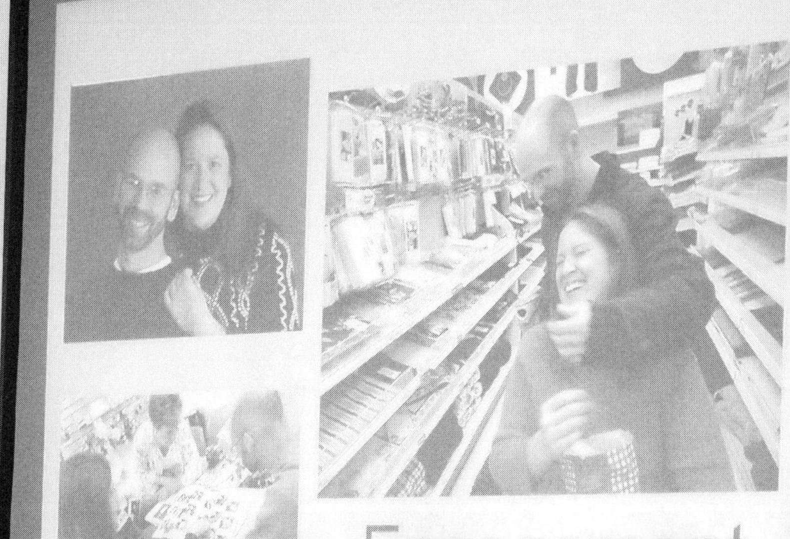

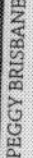

PEGGY BRISBANE

Blessings counted ... even in the bathroom

BY DAN

It was early in the morning, and I was ready to leave for work. A travel mug full of black coffee in my left hand; car keys in my right.

Jennifer rolled down the hallway and asked, "Hey, Dan? Would you have time to help me go to the bathroom one more time before you leave?"

And so I stopped, set my coffee and keys on the floor next to my briefcase, and met her in the bathroom.

As we prepared to make the transfer from her power wheelchair, Jennifer looked up at me and asked, "Do you ever get tired of me always asking you to help me go to the bathroom and all the other stuff you do to help me?"

It certainly wasn't the first time she's asked me such a question, but this time I had a more descript response than my standard reply of, "Never. Do you ever get tired of all the stuff you do to help me?"

I then knelt down to get eye level with Jennifer and asked her if she remembered the time back in 2002, just after we started dating, that I drove back to Iowa by myself for Thanksgiving. And so, there in the bathroom, I shared with Jennifer what had consumed my mind for that 18-hour roundtrip drive to Monticello, Iowa, and back to Mount Pleasant, Mich., some seven years ago.

Imagine that: A tender moment, in the bathroom.

I told Jennifer that for the entire trip I searched for answers to my questions of whether such a relationship could work between two people with MS. Was I going to be strong enough to care for her as well as for myself? Was she going to be strong enough to care for me as well as herself? I threw around the reality that she no longer could walk, and Lord knows how my disease was going to treat me in the future.

It was early enough in our relationship that I think we could have mutually agreed a marriage likely could prove to be more than either of us could handle and MS would force us to "just be friends."

When I returned from Iowa, I had made my decision, and unless Jennifer felt otherwise, I wasn't happy with just being friends.

Fast-forward to 2009, and it was at that moment, in the bathroom, that I fully realized I am living the answers to the questions and prayers I had contemplated on that trip to the Hawkeye State.

I told Jennifer, "On that trip to Iowa, this is what I prayed for: that one day I'd be so blessed as to have you as my wife and we both would be healthy enough that I would be the caregiver for you and you for me, and we didn't let MS prevent us from being happy together. So no, Jennifer, I don't mind at all. This is what I had prayed for."